Power to Heal Opioid and Alcohol Addiction

Recovery Workbook
By Joy Le Page Smith, M.A., BCC

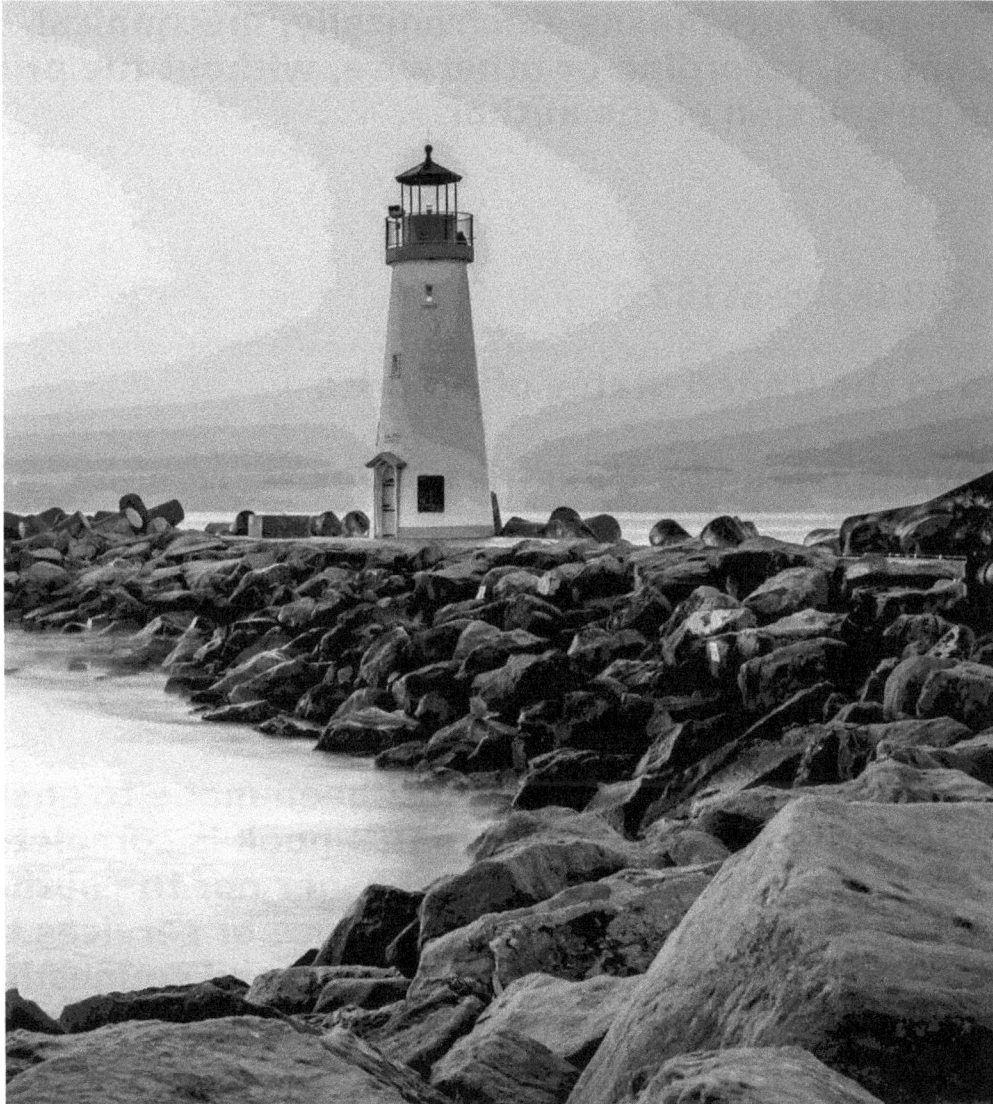

ISBN- 978-0-578-65182-8

Printed in the United States of America

Pathways to Healing – Ministries of Joy

All references used from the Holy Bible are from The New King James version.

Note to the reader: Every effort has been made to ensure that the information contained in this book is complete and accurate. However, neither the publisher nor the author is engaged in rendering professional advice or services to the individual reader. The ideas, procedures and suggestions contained in this book are not intended as a substitute for consulting with your counselor or your physician. All matters regarding your health require medical supervision. Neither the author nor the publisher shall be liable or responsible for any loss, injury or damage allegedly arising from any information or suggestion in this book.

Dedicated

To all who are suffering from addictions —
And to all who are in recovery.

In the dead of night
darkness looms
for those adrift
on a stormy sea.

On the distant horizon –
a lighthouse
illuminating great danger,
unless a change in course.

A brilliant light orients
oneself to safe haven,
fix a respectable distance
avoiding harm's way.

Heave a sigh of relief
for the "darkness felt"
can be cast afar
as you buoy up your inner light.

Gary D. Smith

Foreword

Chaplain Joy is invested and dedicated to creating tools that are meaningful to aid in the path to recovery. Her feelings are palpable through her words guided by a higher power to help those who are ready to rise from rock bottom and be elevated while relearning themselves in recovery.

Lisa Leach, B.S.N., RN
Havasu Regional Medical Center
Director of the Critical Care Service Line
(Sergeant) Retired United States Army

In appreciation to my friends

To my dear husband, Gary Smith, I extend heartfelt gratitude, as without his patience, understanding and loving care this workbook would not be in your hands. I relied heavily on his outstanding language and innate editing skills.

Emily Vona, MSN, FNP-C, took the editing factor of this book to an even higher level of expertise. A heartfelt "thank you" belongs to Emily Vona, and Dr. Leslie Edison. These two medical health providers tutored me regarding the role Medication-assisted- treatment **(MAT),** plays in saving lives. They came alongside in many significant ways. The contributions of Lisa Leach, Director of the Critical Care Service Line, Havasu Regional Medical Center strengthened and polished the work.

It was Dr. Leslie Edison who called to say, "Joy, I am saving lives. And, I need your help." Voile! This workbook! Thank you, Leslie, for being my long term supporter and "inspirer."

I also wholeheartedly thank Pastor Mike Cardello, of Celebrate Recovery and Chery Kitchens, MAPC, Art Therapist. Thank you for your faith in me and in my ability to merge medication, scriptures and a lifestyle philosophy to promote healing helps to those who suffer addiction. To my friend, Mary Jo Mohr, you are a generous soul! Each time I asked you to read, you speedily complied. Many thanks to each of you. I hope you will share the blessing of this book by praying for readers to reach recovery and gain a renewed experience in life.

Table of Contents

A new genesis -- the coming into "being"

David Sheff's book *Beautiful Boy*, presents the sorrow and terror within a father's fight for a son addicted to methamphetamine, who is having perpetual relapses.

"I am in a silent war against an enemy as pernicious and omnipresent as evil. Evil? I don't believe in evil any more than I believe in God. But at the same time I know this: only Satan himself could have designed a disease that has self-deception as a symptom, so that its victims deny they are afflicted, and will not seek treatment, and will vilify those on the outside who see what's happening."[1]

This short quotation of David Sheff reveals it was the drug addiction of his son that opened this father's eyes to one of the worst evils of history. No doubt we cannot believe in a devil without also coming to believe "there is a God" (or "Higher Power," if you prefer).

This workbook is written with a deep and wide belief in God— acknowledging that both good and evil powers are engaged and present on our planet. My intent is to carefully respect the beliefs of all readers while majorly focusing on their struggle against addictions. What I know is that God takes us just as we are.

Superb goodness is seen in our world. And, powerfully so within the fact there is amazing medical help available, along with plenty of easy-to-access informational resources. We must do all

---

[1]Sheff, David. "A Father's Fight for His Son," Special Time Edition, the Science of Addiction What We Know. What We're Learning. Book Excerpt: Meredith Corporation: NY (2019) p. 68.

we can toward putting an end to the current opioid crisis and the growing magnitude of heavy alcohol usage. It is time for all of us to do what we can to address these dreadful circumstances full in the face.

Another "good" to come will be confronting the stigma surrounding both mental illness and substance abuse that keeps addiction in the shadows—and stops people from being honest about needing treatment! Much can be done—and needs to happen speedily—as addictions to alcohol and to opioids are often connected to untreated mental health conditions, such as anxiety and depression.

The reason the opioid epidemic is newsworthy is because so many fatalities are taking place when people use and relapse—and also from intentional suicides due to intense angst that comes from living with a mental health problem or an addiction.

This workbook includes considerable emotional and spiritual help, but purposes to begin with *life-saving information first and foremost*. Again, your best help in achieving recovery from addiction is to seek a medical provider in your area that prescribes medication-assisted treatment (**MAT)**. This zip locator will list health providers in your area: **https://findtreatment.gov/**

This is an approach that combines medications with counseling and other behavioral therapies to treat patients with substance use disorder (SUD). **MAT** blocks the cravings and helps with symptoms of withdrawal for both opioid and alcohol addiction. A more normal life with meaningful work can result. The FDA has approved Medication-assisted treatment and **MAT** is covered by most insurance!

A personalized treatment plan ideally includes counseling and therapy. Counseling will further assist you in building strong coping skills for managing pain, and emotional stress. With this help, you will grow in your ability to set boundaries with yourself and others. Your relationship skills will expand; life will not just be easier—it can become joyous.

No one can doubt that gaining recovery is one of the most difficult challenges. Yet the results are wondrous! It will be like the creation of "new life."

It's all about healing

There will be many opportunities for interactive journaling within the various segments of this workbook. The results you achieve by responding to the questions posed will most likely astound you.

Certainly, recovery is the goal. And, _your determination_ coupled with the help of God (or, "Higher Power") can bring the miracle of becoming the "who," the "what," the "how" and the "when" as you grow into the person you truly want to be. Herein lies potential for you having the kind of life in which you formerly could only dream.

Healing power is at hand, it will come from within you. So, set your goal to complete this workbook. This will initiate a new genesis of self. At the very least this effort will bring:

1) The pleasure of discovering your worth—the goodness within yourself and the "treasure of you" that can enrich the lives of others.

2) Discovering greater potential for health and freedom.

3) Gains a thorough understanding of yourself . . . while seeing clearly what your inner hungers are about.

4) A certainty that you will find _that person you truly desire_ to _be_.

KEY POINT: Get support for the journey. Mike Cardello, Director of the Celebrate Recovery team at Hilltop Church in Lake Havasu City, Ariz., who calls himself "an addict" [recovered], urges "You need an 'accountability team,' meaning 'better together." Mike adds, "Keep in mind, too, that individuals who invest in recovery work grant themselves opportunity to develop rich and rewarding friendships. _But, be cautious! Seek friendships only with people who are sober, not using drugs or alcohol for pain needs or pleasure." Mike also offers this_ encouragement, "Always remember you are not alone. And, that your 'stuff' is not unique."

The best tool I have within my counseling practice (meaning what people are most often thankful for) is to always include God as I work with individuals. I discover what their understanding is of God (or Higher Power). Their intake paperwork includes a release to sign, assuring them that "God will be part of this work." Even atheists have signed that agreement and have done well within my practice. I always hope to introduce people to Christ. Sometimes that happens and often it does not. Yet, within both this workbook and in counseling I purpose to remain where people are most comfortable in respect of this very important fulcrum of life.

The story of your addiction and how it all began

Write about when you started using an addictive substance. Include what was happening in your life at the time:___

Why did you decide to start in the first place:____

When did you know it was an addiction and something you couldn't stop? ____

When did using become a problem for you?____

(More space for writing)

Please write as much as you want or as little as you want. This work is exclusively yours, for your benefit only. No one needs to see your workbook, unless you choose to make exceptions by sharing it with another person.

If you wish to write more about your history with opioid or alcohol use, please do so, filling as many pages as you wish. Write until your soul feels finished.

This is YOUR story!

Thank you for the honesty and the trust you are giving to your recovery!

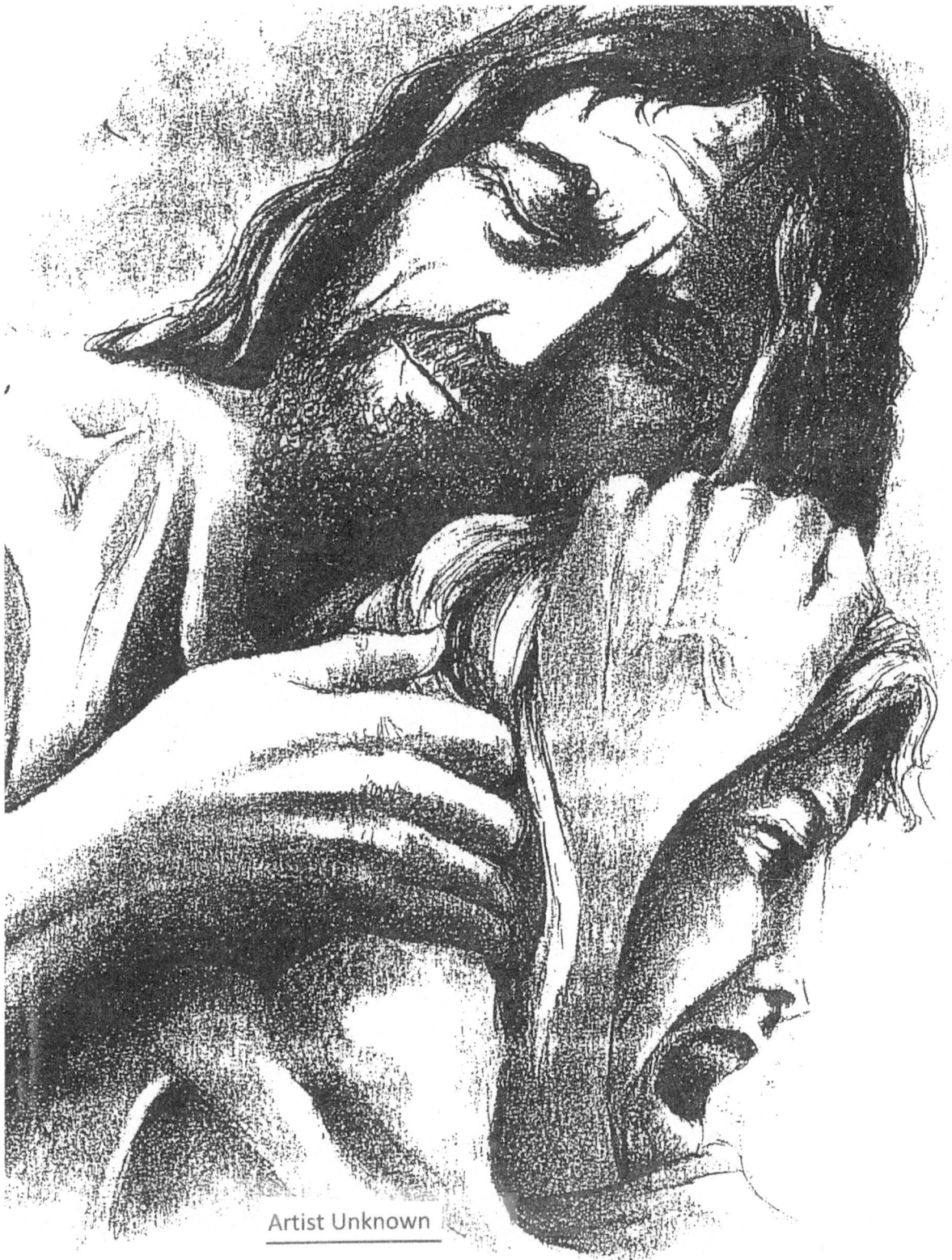

Artist Unknown

About regrets

We all have regrets—perhaps many. It is helpful to write about what you regret most about addiction. Please only write about one, if you write, here. Finish this sentence:

My greatest regret about addiction is:___

(More space for writing)

From here, the best way to work with regrets and making amends—where possible—is to join either the AA 12 Steps Program, the NA 12 Steps program, or attend Celebrate Recovery meetings. Being with others while working through this difficult aspect of addiction recovery brings great benefits. One such benefit is that you will not be doing this work in isolation—you will feel "joined."

If you aren't ready for a group, you can also work through the 12 steps on the Internet. Here are two such sites:

Alcohol.org

help.lionrockrecovery.com

Key point: We all have regrets. You are not alone in your journey.

A new beginning!

Let hope arise! Completing this workbook will bring amazing empowerment for gaining the help you are seeking. Please do not stop this work until you have finished the entire workbook, as doing so will effectively support your desire to get free from your addiction.

Attaining a "new beginning" calls for determination. The resource you hold in your hands will see you caring more deeply about yourself. You will be able to identify the goals you want to reach, while learning techniques for handling your own emotions. Achieving this work will powerfully motivate your resolve to recover from addiction.

If at points you begin feeling "well" and are tempted to lay the workbook aside, refuse to do that. Keep going.

Identifying personal goals: (Check as many as you like.)

☐ Less depression

☐ Less anxiety

☐ Grow spiritually

☐ Gain better coping skills

☐ Increased self-esteem

☐ Feeling I belong

☐ No longer feeling like "I must earn my space (be somebody)"

☐ Feeling safe

☐ Feeling loved

☐ Feeling financially stable

☐ I want to learn how to forgive *who and what* hurts in life

☐ Reach full recovery

☐ Find amazing new friendships

☐ Find what my passion is

☐ For my life to become a pleasure, an adventure

☐ Be able to trust myself

Write anything below that you find missing in the above:

Know yourself better, for good self-care

Finish these sentences.

Why do you think we are here on earth?___

(For help discovering what you want to say about this, see brief article on page 89.)

What do you believe about life?___ (This could pertain to your religious preferences, or to the philosophy you live by.)

In a paragraph (or more) finish this sentence:

I hope for:___

List what you love___ (including "tacos and dogs") ☺

What has been the hardest part of your life?___ (Both past and present, if you wish.)

One of the hardest parts of my life began 26 years ago resulting in a challenge that was bigger than I was. My decision to become a clinical chaplain brought many changes. I signed up for what is called Clinical Pastoral Education, a year-long commitment in a 650 bed teaching hospital. I would be living away from home. The work meant I would be seeing and experiencing things that would pierce my heart over and over again.

There were nine of us who dedicated ourselves to serve in this way. We rotated with each of us being on-call alone for 24 hours every 9th day. My first trauma was an eight year old boy who got up from the dinner table, took his father's gun, went outside in the yard, knelt before a friend and said, "I don't want to go to school tomorrow." Then this child shot himself in the heart. I stood at his head and watched—praying—as the medical team did everything possible to save his life. Regardless, he died. About halfway into my year-long chaplaincy training I was in the trauma center of this Phoenix hospital when I wrote on a scrap of paper in pencil; I will call it "A Chaplain's cry for help."

Lord, where are you?
You are here, I know . . .
But, I'm grasping to take ahold;
I'm losing my grip.
The gunman saved today
Will be on the streets tomorrow.
I'm saturated with the trauma,
The drug deaths, the senseless shootings.
Where are you, Lord? What help, am I,
A chaplain at their bedsides?
"My child, I am here. I am in the shooter.
I am in the dealer. I am in the user . . .
In the very breath they breathe.
Pray for my release. I await, there,
As your prayers are what I need."

God is a seeker of hearts, desiring to become a part of our lives through prayer; He wants us to make our decisions in a way that blesses us and blesses others. We are the Beloved of our Creator who will not ask more of us than we are able to give. His support will provide strength and empowerment to help us become all we can be in this life.

Depression and anxiety

Depression is felt when we feel sad to the point of losing interest in the things that we have enjoyed in the past. When we are depressed, we feel bad and hardly anything seems appealing. This is a mood disorder that affects what we think, what we feel and how we behave. Depression can cause us to miss opportunities and play havoc with our relationships. It can affect our decisions and adversely influence friendships. Depression is "the pits."

Lisa Firestone, Ph.D, writes, "People who suffer from depression often have intense '**critical inner voices**' that perpetuate feelings of unworthiness and **shame**. When we listen to this **inner critic**, we not only feel more depressed, but may also find it much more difficult to stand up to the depression . . . **Sigmund Freud** used to refer to **depression** as **anger** turned inward. While many people may regard this as an overly simplistic approach to the most common mental health disorder in the world, there is no doubt that anger plays a significant role in depression. As one study from 2016 found, when it comes to emotional disorders in general, the presence of anger has negative consequences, including greater symptom severity and worse treatment response."[2]

Do you recognize what Dr. Firestone says about "critical inner voices"?

Yes___   No___

Describe: How do you handle anger?

Circle the number that best applies:

1) Gulp it down and fume;

---

[2] Firestone, Lisa. "The Role of Anger in Depression," https://www.Psychologytoday.com/us/blog/compassion-matters/201710/the-role-anger-in-depression. (Accessed, February 21, 2020.)

2) turn it against yourself;

3) spew it out in angry words;

4) wait for a chance to get even;

5) handle it with an "I feel statement" (e.g., "I hurt when you stayed out all night without calling.")

The upside down diagram on the next page shows how anger can be used to look deeper and discover the fear that is underneath the anger. It also shows how anger can help us get real about what's actually hurting us. When we are angry we also have hurt. And, when we have hurt, we have anger. Beneath these emotions is fear. Healing comes when we look at the fear beneath these emotions. "Find the fear— and let go of the fear." In life, it is important to understand the dynamics taking place within ourselves when we experience emotions.

Work with the following diagram when desiring to handle anger, hurt and fear in a healthy way.

It takes some persistence to learn the above pattern, as it is a new way of being. Always remember: "If you fail once, it does not mean you fail always."

The Upside down triangle

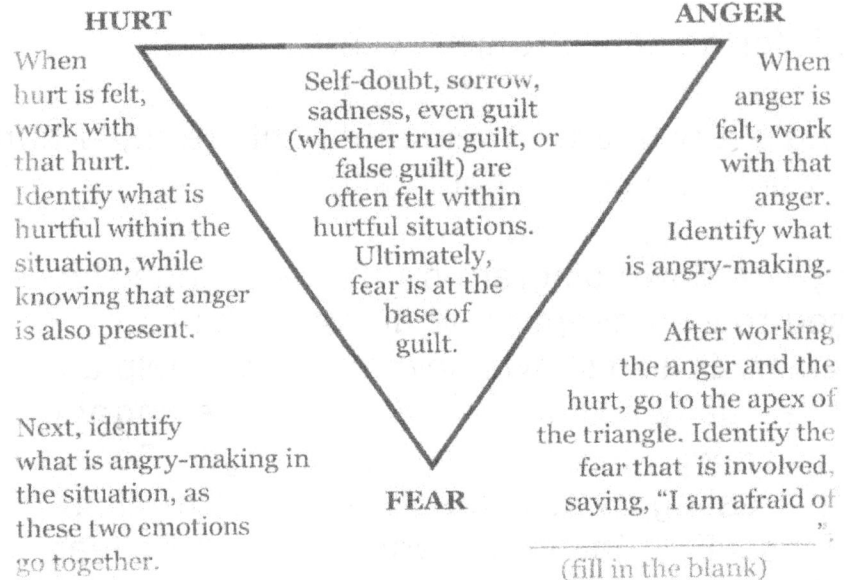

HURT   **ANGER**

When hurt is felt, work with that hurt. Identify what is hurtful within the situation, while knowing that anger is also present.

Self-doubt, sorrow, sadness, even guilt (whether true guilt, or false guilt) are often felt within hurtful situations. Ultimately, fear is at the base of guilt.

When anger is felt, work with that anger. Identify what is angry-making.

After working the anger and the hurt, go to the apex of the triangle. Identify the fear that is involved, saying, "I am afraid of

_____."

Next, identify what is angry-making in the situation, as these two emotions go together.

FEAR

(fill in the blank)

Anger is sometimes felt when we are frustrated. It, at times, accompanies disappointment—even embarrassment and confusion. Honoring and identifying feelings can definitely help with self-understanding. Most researchers agree that by age six, a person's belief system is reasonably well formed.[1] Distinguishing emotions, as they arise, can help a person discover early perceptions and beliefs held throughout life regarding the world, God—and what is right, what is wrong. This can bring clarity as to when boundaries with others are needed and warranted. Besides these personal gains, this work can pave the way for observing some "ancient" beliefs that may need to be re-examined in order to fit life as a growing adult.

---

[1] Larisa Heiphetz,[a] Elizabeth S. Spelke,[b] Paul L. Harris,[c] and Mahzarin R. Banaji[d] The Development of Reasoning about Beliefs: Fact, Preference, and Ideology, https://www.ncbi.nlm.nih.gov/pmc/articles/PMC3667744/ (Oct 13, 2012)

(More space for writing)

It is clear that repressed anger and sadness can play a significant role prolonging depression, at times, even causing it. Talking or journaling about anger and sadness helps to release the pain. This way you are not holding it all in. In the Addendum section of this workbook you will find an article on tears. This article carries a medical doctor's understanding of how crying can actually help our bodies. Our bodies need to release a chemical that builds up when we are stressed. Tears carries that build up away when we cry. Think of it as cleansing. (See page 93 in the Addendum.)

Has depression been part of your life during recent years?

Yes____

No_____

If yes, has this been a persistent problem throughout your life?___

Or, does depression come and go?__

Here, write all that you want to about your experiences with depression.__

(More space for writing)

Describe the hurt of depression—what does it feel like when it comes?

What percentage of your life do you estimate that depression has been a major influence?___

What is the greatest loss you have experienced in your life due to depression?___

(More space for writing)

Some say, "If you don't deal with your emotions, your emotions will deal with you." This is true—and especially true of repressed anger. Some of us hold anger—as well as hurt and fear—inside. We gulp these down instead of knowing how to express them. Often, showing our emotions is considered a sign of weakness. That forces us to push them way down inside, pretending they are gone.

Lisa Firestone, Ph.D., says it well, "Many of the people I've worked with who struggle with depression also share the common struggle of turning their anger on themselves. As much as I try to help my clients express their anger rather than take it on and turn it inward, I witness first-hand how hard it often is for people to interrupt this process. It's a challenge for them to recognize the nasty way they treat themselves; they are significantly more critical of themselves than they are of others."[3]

You may ask, "How can I stand against depression?" By identifying the good in yourself and knowing this goodness is your truth. Acting against those critical inner voices, caused by anger turned inward, will include taking positive actions that help you

---

[3] Firestone, Lisa. "The Role of Anger in Depression," https://www.Psychologytoday.com/us/blog/compassion-matters/201710/the-role-anger-in-depression. (Accessed, February 21, 2020.)

feel better about yourself. For sure, it takes courage to push past depression and reach out to a friend or neighbour.

You have every right to care about yourself. Try choosing an enjoyable activity or pastime to share with another person. As Lisa Firestone puts it, "Being more social in life can be a powerful aid against depression. It takes courage to be honest with ourselves and others, saying, "I need help. Would you please help me get through this?"[4]

Depression and anxiety are often experienced together. When depressed, we know something very big is amiss in our lives. So, this scares us. Life seems uncertain. It is hard to find out what causes the worry that accompanies so much of our thoughts. Sometimes panic attacks take place when apprehension is great. This can be so strong we think we are having a heart attack. The good news: the panic attacks <u>can be stopped!</u>

A person with anxiety may study the signs of a panic attack to learn more and become aware of how to stop one before it is experienced.

Eleven ways to stop a panic attack can be found at: **https://www.healthline.com/health/how-to-stop-a-panic-attack**

There is absolutely no shame in having depression and/or anxiety. And, certainly there is no shame in experiencing a panic attack. Some people will have times of experiencing both of these difficult moods disorders at some points in life. It is part of being human.

Has anxiety been part of your life?   Yes_____   No_____

---

[4]Firestone, Lisa. "The Role of Anger in Depression," https://www.Psychologytoday.com/us/blog/compassion-matters/201710/the-role-anger-in-depression. (Accessed, February 21, 2020.)

If "Yes" is your response, has anxiety been constant throughout your life, or does it come and go?___

What percentage of your life do you estimate that anxiety has majorly influenced your life?_

Here are three websites that offer help with depression, anxiety and other emotional struggles that interfere with recovery:

www.AZRecover.com

https://psychcentral.com/

https://screening.mhanational.org/screening-tools

At the latter site, Mental Health America extends great opportunities to do self-testing with good tools and your privacy is protected. Go ahead and see for yourself.

Health History

A brain injury can affect behaviour, moods and lead to substance abuse. Check your health history.

For some, traumatic brain injuries (TBIs) happened as early in life as birth or as a baby. If you know or suspect this could be part of your health history, you may gain from viewing Dr. Daniel Amen's Youtube at:

https://www.youtube.com/watch?v=esPRsT-lmw8

Daniel Amen, is a medical doctor who has written several books and designed programs that hold amazing findings as regards brain injuries and what can result from them.

Dr. Amen's book titles include intriguing titles such as, *Change Your Brain Change Your Life* and *Feel Better Fast and Make it Last*. Other books and programs by Amen can be found at:

https://danielamenmd.com/programs-books/

If you have experienced one or more head injuries, record these below:___   (If there were several, include your age with each occurrence.)

List here any ways in which you think your health experience(s) may be affecting your addiction(s):___

Seek and build your support system

There is real value (both emotional and spiritual) in letting others witness your journey. A support group setting allows you to share the happenings of your life while surrounded with people who have compassion—as they know what you are going through. In this setting love has opportunity to flow.

Be sure to find a support group that is sufficient for your goal of good self-care. A support group that includes the help of a power higher than yourself is best of all.

This group will help you identify your own strengths while encouraging others in your group to be self-nurturing. Within the group, each can also safely share what helps with relaxation. (See page 42, for "Building healthy coping skills.") Hobbies, sports and activities can bring fun and excitement to your life in healthy ways.

During my past 25 years of mental health counseling, a tell-tale pattern became clear through observing the intake paper work of hundreds of clients. An absolute recipe for a break down is seen when a person:

* does not know his or her strengths,

* does not have an adequate support system in place, and is

* doing nothing to nurture herself or himself.

Some people look for a solution in alcohol, illegal drugs, and/or inappropriate use of prescription drugs when they know a break down is coming (meaning they feel totally out of control and are greatly afraid). They self-medicate.

Self-medicating is dangerous, both physically and mentally. Instead, contact a medical health provider for treatment. When Medication-assisted-treatment (**MAT**) is included **lives can be saved**. With medication in place, normality can be restored without heading directly into the catastrophe of spiraling downward.

Describe your current support system___ (Please list one or two people who you can trust to talk with, telling anything to that person without fear of betrayal or manipulation.)

It is very important to know you must be selective as to the people you choose to be in relationship with. Ask yourself, "Are they trustworthy? Do they have the same or similar goals as mine? Do they care deeply about my values enough to honor my boundaries?"

Another aspect of selecting who you will trust involves determining if a potential friend self-medicates through "using," or are they choosing to live sober, set meaningful goals and to live a meaningful life?

Who would you like to add to your support team?___

Be sure to <u>be your own best support</u> . . . doing good things for yourself, while also having other supportive people in your life.

List here some good things you are doing to nurture yourself:___ (See page 39,"Building self-esteem for maintaining good self-care." There you will find a list of nurturing activities.)

Do you attend community support meetings, such as AA, NA, or Celebrate Recovery regularly?

☐ Yes ☐ No

If yes, how frequently do you attend?__

If no, please write why not__

Check here if you attend more than one community support group.

Do you attend church? ☐ yes   ☐ no

Do you attend a club, or lodge? ☐ yes   ☐ no

Are you a part of any group activities? ☐ yes   ☐ no

List each current involvement that you find helpful:__

Write here about how past efforts have supported your sobriety__

List your strengths: (If you cannot think of any, ask a trusted friend what she or he sees your strengths to be.) Write these down. Read your list daily—YES! Out loud.

(More space for writing)

Love yourself!

To love one's self is stated by Christ as being an <u>essential part</u> of following the commandments given to us by God:

"'You shall love the L<small>ORD</small> your God with all your heart, with all your soul, and with all your mind.' [38] This is *the* first and greatest commandment. [39] And *the* second *is* like it: 'You shall love your neighbour **as yourself**.' [40] On these two commandments hang all the Law and the Prophets," (Matthew 22: 36-40).[5]

Self-love is far from "being selfish," which involves not caring about the needs of others. Many of the problems within humanity are caused by lacking love for one's self. Failure to love ourselves will see us trying to fill up the emptiness this creates, resulting in addictions of various sorts. For example, overeating—or even overworking or excessive recreation—will not substitute for taking good care of one's self, meeting needs that can only come through making sure we are loving and respecting ourselves.

---

[5] Although this scripture passage is slightly different in other versions, please know the New King James Version is used throughout this workbook.

Building self-esteem for maintaining good self-care

This is a process and can be aided by responding to the following:

Identify the uniqueness of yourself. Include positive things family and friends say about you___ (A later section, at page 63, "Explore your abilities," will help discover these. Write what comes to mind at this time.)

Consider telling yourself the truth, use statements about your strengths (and other positive affirmations) daily-- especially when:

- You are feeling low
- You are having negative thoughts about yourself
- When another person says something hurtful to you

Identify any negative thoughts of yourself that you entertain, or self-criticism. NOW, refuse these. (See "Stop Thought," for a powerful technique, on page 84 within the Addendum of this workbook.)

Have compassion for yourself—be your own best friend.

When complimented by another person, can you say, "Thank you" and consciously receive that truth about yourself? Can you truly take it in, accepting it and believing it?

Yes____

No____

If your answer is no, do you want to practice self-love by changing a pattern of the past?

Yes____

No____

If your answer is "no," list what you think is a belief about yourself that is unloving. Write a belief that you can let go of today:___

Each day, do something that makes you feel good about yourself, like, hiking, biking, enjoying a friendship, finishing a task that is bugging you. <u>Then pat yourself on the back.</u>

Decide today: Are you willing to start loving yourself by doing what you are learning within recovery work—including letting go of dark thoughts about yourself?

Yes____

No____

List any justifiable reason that warrants self-criticism:___

Make it a habit to question it each time you bad-mouth yourself.

You are well on your way. Your dedication to complete this workbook is an act of self-love. Continue doing a few pages as often as possible until finished. Take time to savor, recognize and applaud what you are doing. This is how you save yourself.

Enjoy getting to know yourself better—and learning to love yourself.

Give yourself permission to grow in your ability to **acknowledge your worth**. (See pages 74 and 99, in the Addendum for a list of Biblical passages, encouraging you to build your self-esteem, learn your self-worth—and soothe your soul.)

As you read the passages make notes, here, as regards thoughts which may arise for you:

Building healthy coping skills

Living with addiction means "using" has likely been your coping skill. This was your "most relied on and most desired" means for feeling OK in this world. So, how has that worked for you so far?

This segment of the workbook is intended to help you find new ways to deal with difficult feelings, quiet and calm yourself, and put you in a better place mentally and emotionally thus allowing you to take control of the urgings or cravings. Developing new coping skills will help you learn to endure, reduce and manage situations in life that are difficult and/or highly stressful. You will reach far greater enjoyment in a life that you control and design. This is the result of good self-care.

Foremost: Doing breathing exercises is often a great way to begin your day. Also use deep breathing any time you feel tense or out of sorts. *This is a coping skill*. Teach yourself to use deep breathing as a great and effective tool for easing anxiety and promoting relaxation.

Deep breathing is a mighty coping skill.

It brings oxygen to your brain.

You can do it at any point or place you want to. When you start tensing up (shoulders ache, tongue on the roof of your mouth, jaw clenched), feeling anxious, this is a moment to remember good self-care is in order! Pause. Start breathing deeply, taking in more air. This exercise in breathing strengthens and supports your nervous system resulting in you empowering yourself to remain calm.

Addiction itself is highly stressful. It is <u>an enslavement</u>.

Truth be known, developing coping skills and learning how to set boundaries are the two main ways to control stress on a daily basis. Going forward, your help with these two elements of good self-care will be the focus and will make a remarkable difference in your *health and happiness for your future*.

Finding ways to deal with unexpected things that happen will greatly lessen your stress level. A major element of developing coping skills lies with learning how to take good self-care. Everyone knows what can be fun or enjoyable in life. But when we get sick, we forget what nurtures us, and then fail to take good care of ourselves.

Pick activities from the list below that you want to try as you strategize toward developing (or returning to) a loving friendship with yourself. Discover the comfort of simply being who you are and appreciating what appeals to you. Learn to hold the space of enjoying yourself.

Use the list below during hard times when you feel uncomfortable in your skin, or highly pressured. Even if you only "spark" on one or two of the possibilities, that will be great. It is a place to start.

The first two on this list are coping skills on record for having been highly effective for many people through the ages.

- Meditation and/or prayer

- Read Holy Writ while listening for what soothes your heart

- Exercise using gym equipment, or other methods like biking

- Take a walk, ideally 30-40 minutes; or a run, based on the state
    of your health

- Visit a pet shelter (where you can talk to and pet animals)

- Use a relaxation app or practice progressive muscle relaxation

- Listen to music, or play a musical instrument

- Sing or hum at points when anxiety arises or you feel depressed

- Make a blessing or gratitude list ("I am thankful for . . . ")

- Enjoy water (swimming, soaking bath, or by other means)

- Talk to yourself (journaling is a meaningful way to do this)

- Pop bubble wrap (larger size)—popping them with your fingers as you think of what you are angry about. Release the difficult feelings as you do the pop the bubble

- Draw, color, paint, sculpt, or do ceramics

 - Play with a pet, or a friend's pet

- Try a new recipe, then ask friends, "come over to help eat"

- Clean a messy drawer, cabinet or closet that has been
      bothering you

- Take a drive . . . find a nature path to explore

- Read your favorite kind of book

- Enjoy playing cards with a friend, or friends, e.g.,
      Bunco, spades, hand and foot

- Plan time with friends or family who have a baby; rock the baby

- Spend time with friends or family who have kids. Play games
      like a kid

- Look into a new hobby

- Look at landscape photos that help you feel relaxed

- Go to a park just to listen and watch what all takes place there

- Visit a zoo, science display, or museum

- Go to your favorite type of movie (or see one on a device)

- Visit a skating arena; watch and join in, if physically able

- Dance!

- List good times and blessed events of your life

- List all for which you are thankful

- Sit by the water—breath, listen, smell and look around

- Ask a loved one to rub your shoulders . . . or, go get a massage

- Laugh as often as you can—even to pretend laughter (it works)

- Google funny Youtube videos, e.g. my favorite is:

   https://www.youtube.com/watch?v=b2qM1I-JCEQ

- Google Youtube sing-along videos

- Take some time in a shopping center; watch and listen to enjoy

- Pursue something you want to learn about; share with a friend

- Ride a bike or skate as often as possible

- Look at people while giving a smile; watch their eyes: enjoy!

- Find a contemplative water fountain (or waterfall in nature) --

   sit and listen to the H20

-      Listen to Ted Talks to get your mind completely off of everything.

Also consider Ted Talks at **https://www.ted.com/talks**. There are many youtube videos on various subjects that will grab your full attention, put you in a different "space"—and are likely to even challenge your thinking.

Remember, moving your body in challenging ways and fully occupying your mind will put you in a different space. Try it.

Here are some places to go to switch gears, in order to reach a more relaxing, more joyful "space":

These youtube videos will do wonders with putting you in "good space."

https://www.youtube.com/watch?v=75PUjUsGsQQ (takes only 2 minutes)

https://www.youtube.com/watch?v=XUKrtkHbA90 (minutes of fun dance)

https://www.youtube.com/watch?v=UxOpnhY6ObU

(pictures with music; 5 ½ minutes)

Now, return to the list of coping skills. Circle each entry above that is something that piques your interest, or is an activity you have enjoyed in the past.

Then write below indicating which of these coping skills you will want to begin using, during times when you feel so uncomfortable that you are tempted to use.___

Dr. Nora Vocci, director of the National Institute of Drug Abuse states that stress alters the way the brain thinks, "The part of the prefrontal cortex that is involved in deliberative cognition is shut down by stress."[6] So, enjoy as many of the above stress reducing activities as you can—and as often as you can. This will help you

---

[6] Lemonick, Michael. The Science of Addiction. *Special Time Edition, the Science of Addiction What We Know. What We're Learning.* Book Excerpt: Meredith Corporation: NY (2019) p. 8.

minimize stress. This will help guard against making impulsive choices.

Reaching recovery and maintaining it will take diligence and hard work. Medication-assisted-treatment (**MAT**), prayer and this workbook, along with your support group meetings, can see you reaching your goal of achieving recovery. If you are not in a support group, please consider getting into one—or, at least stay close to your "support people."

List them here:___

Setting boundaries

Learning to set boundaries with yourself and for others is among the most powerful of all coping skills. This skill, if practiced consistently will change the dynamics of all your relationships—for the good, allowing for less stress in life. Stress, as we know, affects our health mentally, physically and emotionally. Consequently, this is the longest segment of the workbook. Yet, it will bring knowledge that holds potential for reaping great benefits.

Certainly, it takes great courage, persistence and discernment to develop abilities that support you doing well in life. Learning to set and maintain boundaries with self and others takes awareness of the various "Types of boundaries" in which feelings, thoughts and values need to be honored. These are identified by Margarita Tartakovsky, M.S. at Psych Central as:

"**Material boundaries** determine whether you give or lend things, such as your money, car, clothes, books, food, or toothbrush.

"**Physical boundaries** pertain to your personal space, privacy, and body. Do you give a handshake or a hug – to whom and when? How do you feel about loud music, nudity, and locked doors?

"**Mental boundaries** apply to your thoughts, values, and opinions. Are you easily suggestible? Do you know what you believe, and can you hold onto your opinions? Can you listen with an open mind to someone else's opinion without becoming rigid? If you become highly emotional, argumentative, or defensive, you may have weak emotional boundaries.

"**Emotional boundaries** distinguish separating your emotions and responsibility from someone else's. It's like an imaginary line or force field that separates you and others. Healthy boundaries prevent you from giving advice, blaming or accepting blame. They protect you from feeling guilty for someone else's negative feelings or problems and taking others' comments personally. High reactivity suggests weak emotional boundaries. Healthy emotional boundaries require clear internal boundaries – knowing your feelings and your responsibilities to yourself and others.

"**Sexual boundaries** protect your comfort level with sexual touch and activity – what, where, when, and with whom.

"**Spiritual boundaries** relate to your beliefs and experiences in connection with God or a higher power." [7]

Write a paragraph or more about a current situation(s) or relationship in which you need to set boundaries: __

Write how it feels to set a boundary, then find it is not honored:__

Can you think of a time when you did not honor someone else's boundaries? If so, write a sentence or two about how that felt for you, after the fact:__

---

[7]Tartakovsky. Margarita, "10 Way to Build and Preserve Better Boundaries," *Psych Central*, https://psychcentral.com/lib/10-way-to-build-and-preserve-better-boundaries/ (Accessed February 13, 2020.) Copyright 2020 PsychCentral.com. All rights reserved. Reprinted here with permission.

(More space for writing)

You already know that you must set boundaries with yourself in order to achieve recovery. This is important—and equally so with others making sure they honor your boundaries. You can truly live your own life and respect yourself on a new level. By knowing what you want in your relationships and setting clear boundaries but the rewards will be great!

Prior to having a conversation about a boundary that needs to be set, or honored, carefully choose the words that will best describe your goal. If fear or anxiety begins to set in, do deep breathing for a moment or two. Then state the boundary you need with this person. Next, stipulate a **consequence** for the person in the event your boundary is not respected. Without consequences, your boundaries will be ignored.

For example, imagine a time when you were stood up by a person you were dating. Decide what behavior you want them to change and be clear. Your boundary statement must be strong, "I don't want to be stood up again." This stipulates what you need. Add, "...regardless of how hard this will be for me—I will not continue going out with you." Now, a boundary has been set along with a consequence. Always be open and caring, wanting to hear a response. This can be a learning experience for both of you. Listen for understanding—before responding. An attitude of caring, coupled with good listening skills, goes a long way within good relationships.

Be prepared, your boundaries will be tested. Stand your ground. In the instance above, the person could ask for another date. You then can show a firm stance by using words that mean business. For instance, "I cannot trust a person who does not respect my boundaries."

Relationships are heavily involved with feelings. Honoring your feelings will necessitate doing some work to determine where these feelings are coming from.

KEY POINT: Feelings don't just happen. Feelings follow thoughts! "The Motivational Model" (author unknown) on the following page portrays this truth and shows the importance of what we believe and how we perceive.

Confrontation with others can involve some intense feelings. The key to success during confrontation is to modulate these three aspects of your communication: manner, timing, and intensity. Tone of voice used is a factor that makes a huge difference. These are elements of speech over which you have control. Sometimes, we lose a relationship. Growth comes in learning from the experience. Within healthy relationships, it is almost always possible to work through difficulties as they arise, providing each party is willing to keep caring, keep talking.

Here is a powerful tool to use in life (and I, too, am working on it): Stop caring what others think of you. Beyond working on your relationships in caring ways, tell yourself, "**What others think of me is none of my business**." Using the Stop thought" technique on page 84 of the Addendum, as needed, will make this possible. And, this brings a specific empowerment.

Doing our best to live a healthy, loving life, while doing what we can to be productive, is a powerful way to be in the world. It grants empowerment to just **be who we are**. Making the best choices we can day-by-day, while learning from our mistakes, having every reason for holding good thoughts about ourselves.

The Motivational Model

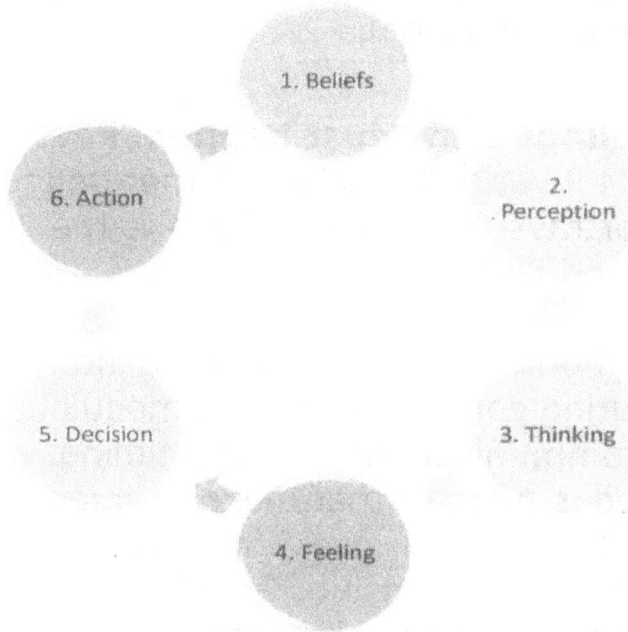

1. Beliefs

2. Perception

6. Action

3. Thinking

5. Decision

4. Feeling

What most people do not know:

Our beliefs create our perceptions

    * how we see the world, ourselves, God and others

Our perceptions create our thoughts

Our thoughts create our feelings

Our feelings largely influence our decisions

Our decisions create our actions

Our actions either reinforce our beliefs or help

us change our beliefs.

Become keenly aware of when your boundaries are breached, disrespected, ignored.

Rule of thumb: If something (said or done) *"feels like* a kick in the stomach—*it's probably a kick in the stomach*." Here is some help with addressing that "kick."

1) When something said to you feels unfair or disrespectful, you have the right to ask the person to restate their meaning.

2) Don't be afraid to share your thoughts and your feelings when words said don't feel fair or fitting. It works best to answer with an *"I feel statement*." For example, "Right now I feel hurt." (Or, "I feel punished, treated like a child, misunderstood, put down or disrespected.)

3) Open with strength. With the above scenario of saying, "I feel hurt." Think of it as if you're playing tennis and you have just sent that "I feel statement" like a ball into the other person's court. Then that person whacks the ball back to you, saying, "Well, now *you* know what it feels like to be hurt. What you said *to me* the other day was rude."

You can ask a question to get the ball moving again, like, "Are you saying you think I have bad manners—or are you saying I have done something that has embarrassed, or hurt you?"
This allows clarification. The goal, here, is for both parties to gain understanding. When fairness rules, *both parties* want resolution. Do not interrupt. Rather, listen to understand the person.

When a person stays in the game, clarification comes and some understanding can be gained. It becomes easy to admit what you may need to own up to—and likewise for the other person to do the same. Apologies are certainly easier to make when both see their role and can be honest, able to accept what part she or he has played in the problem.

If you can keep the conversation going, there is hope for the two of you to reach whatever it is that threatens your relationship. This will take reining in your feelings, express them carefully, caring as much about the other person as you do for yourself. This is a powerful way of being in the world. It works exceedingly well when desiring to resolve a problem.

Another rule of thumb: If you do not feel safe within a conversation--***STOP***. Choose **another time and place** to have the discussion you want, or need to have with this person. It is OK to say, "I need space for now. We can choose to talk about this again later." (Here, you are setting a boundary.)

When you need to talk about something that is bothersome, it works best to simply begin with, "I have felt bothered about something." Be prepared to *listen* while the person responds. *Reflecting back* what you've heard helps to avoid any misunderstandings. Being fully honest and hearing one another are the keys to solving a problem and setting a boundary.

Setting boundaries and maintaining them is all about taking good care of ourselves. It takes time and ongoing efforts to develop this skill. It is wise to take the advice of psychologist and coach, Dr. Dana Giota, "Build upon your success, and [at first] try not to take on something that feels overwhelming."[8]

People who are highly developed, and even those who are just beginning to work on themselves, *will respect your boundaries when these are clearly set—even when they do not like doing so.* This is the kind of friend you will want to add into your life.

A major aspect of setting boundaries lies with realizing the importance of feelings. Identify your feelings and honor them.

---

[8]Tartakovsky. Margarita. "10 Way to Build and Preserve Better Boundaries, Psych Central, https://psychcentral.com/lib/10-way-to-build-and-preserve-better-boundaries/ (Accessed February 13, 2020.) Copyright 2020 PsychCentral.com. All rights reserved. Reprinted here with permission.

Doing so is a huge part of growing, *then maintaining* strong self-awareness and appreciation. (If you don't have these for yourself, no one else will.)

Essential elements of boundary-setting:

- Trusting yourself means trusting your feelings.

  - Give yourself permission to deal with your most difficult feelings. A common practice is to swallow—gulp down—these feelings. But honoring and identify them will help you get well and prepare you for setting boundaries with other people.

- Identify what it is that you are feeling. Are you feeling mad? Are you feeling sad? Or, are you feeling glad? Are you feeling afraid? Disappointed? Frustrated? Are you feeling betrayed? Or, are you feeling guilty? Confused?

  Rick Warren, who started the powerfully effective 12 step program Celebrate Recovery with John Baker in 1991, succinctly says, "Revealing the feeling is the beginning of healing."[9]

- Determine what your feelings are saying. Feelings often hold a message. *Listen* for the message. This is a skill to develop.

Honor and identify your feelings:

In a paragraph (or more) finish these sentences:

Ponder feeling(s), <u>not</u> thoughts, as you answer this: What I **feel** most at this time in life is:___

---

[9] https://www.crosswalk.com/devotionals/daily-hope-with-rick-warren/daily-hope-with-rick-warren-june-19-2016.html (Accessed January 7, 2020).

(More space for writing)

What I find myself **thinking about** most, presently is:___

I think positively on a daily basis: Yes_____ no_____

I think negatively: yes_____ no_____

If you think negatively as a pattern, do you want to change this?
yes____ no____

Thinking positively will find you seeing your life differently. A practice of noticing and owning all for which you can be thankful will create "happy hormones" (endorphin flows). In time, this will lead to you feeling up more than you are feeling down. Voila! Fewer low moods or depression—therefore, less anxiety. A close look at a field of medicine, psychoneuroimmunology (PNI), will reveal how your body responds to what you are thinking and believing. Therefore, whatever is going on in your psyche (soul) affects your immune system, neurological system and hormonal system. (The National Institute of Health is an excellent resource for facts on PNI.)

KEY POINT: "We are not responsible for anyone else's feelings. We *are* responsible for choosing to be considerate of the feelings of others—while also being considerate of our own feelings."[10]

Practice assertiveness so you can best succeed with boundary setting. Within a conflict, speak calmly in your natural tone of

---

[10] Author unknown. A quotation in Ottawa U. class notes.

voice—and speak with care. Say what you want to take place, meaning say what you need. Then, if you don't feel heard and the conversation does not stay on track, make that same statement, again. This serves well with holding boundaries in place.

When serious matters that affect relationships need discussing, some conversations are best done in public, for instance in a restaurant where other people are close by. **If any sense of danger is felt, trust your intuition.** It could be an appropriate time for a minister, priest or a mediator to be involved. Some matters call for legal action in order to be settled safely and fairly. Never, never, never live, work or be in unsafe conditions.

Boundary setting is not about "getting your way." It is about being in healthy relationships within life. This is how we can have a much better existence while here on earth. Those who have not learned how to be in an enriching relationship are more apt to yield to the temptation to use alcohol or other mind-altering substances to try to escape a nasty reality.

Few people are taught that they *have a right* to set boundaries. Therefore, few people know how to set or maintain boundaries. Yet, hardly anyone can have strong, lasting relationships without knowing how to do good self-care. Clearly, frequent overuse of alcohol and drugs comes from people who are out of touch with themselves and not knowing any of the elements of loving one's self. Hoping for a quick fix they often self-medicate with substances that are harmful. They may not believe that there is a better way.

Seeing a counselor or a mental health practitioner is the way many people first learn about their right to set boundaries and to stipulate consequences when their boundaries are not respected and honored. Frequently good-self-care training only comes for people after a breakdown—or after a person finds herself or himself in substance abuse/addiction.

The skill of boundary setting will increase through determining to _let the fear go_! _Fear of making someone unhappy can feel intimidating. But, loving yourself means living courageously_. Doing so means we seriously seek the ability to feel and to express what is going on. We accept where we have been—and where we are going. We set goals. This puts us in a good place for lovingly serving our own needs in healthy ways.

For me, this meant going back to school at age 60 to gain the credentials needed to do the work of my heart. I now feel superbly blessed working as a clinical chaplain, serving people who are sick, dying or otherwise in deep trouble. I can understand what Jesus Christ meant in calling the people in need "the least of these my brethren."

Dr. Carl Jung put a unique spin on this: "What if I should discover that the least of all brethren,[11] the poorest of all beggars, the most insolent of all offenders, yes, even the very enemy himself—that these live within me; that I myself stand in need of the alms of my own kindness, that I am to myself the enemy who is to be loved?"

This takes us back to our challenge of becoming able to identify and cherish the true essence _of ourselves_. Now, real hope for recovery takes place. This work of validating and loving ourselves will act as a springboard moving us speedily and spontaneously toward truly "be-ing," respecting our passion and our visions as these develop.

Loving myself seemed impossible. My parents did not say, "I love you" while growing up. I also do not remember their speaking any terms of endearment. What is for sure, is they were good, hard working dam-construction and farming people who provided

---

[11]Mathew 25:40, "And the King will answer and say to them, 'Assuredly, I say to you, inasmuch as you did _it_ to one of the least of these My brethren, you did _it_ to Me.'"

for the needs of their children. They honored their parents. By mid-life my mother and father became influential, helping many people by becoming teachers of "the Way," meaning the teachings of Christ. I was raised by then. God's presence was at work, growing in them. I could see they truly loved others; it was obvious—easily seen through how they served others. But, for me, there was a sense of feeling less than loveable. I always felt I wasn't quite enough . . . needing to be more than I was.

The truth that *God loves me*—for myself, as I am—became possible from reading the Bible cover to cover. This revealed the Creator's love *as fact, not fiction*. (In the Addendum, on page 85, you will find a shortcut for finding God's love as you read "The Cry of Our Father's Heart" where words paraphrased from the Holy Bible—from the books of Genesis through Revelation—reveal how we are loved.)

Coming to love one's self brings many strengths. We come to be at peace with ourselves—"warts and all." We find joy and valor. We become enabled to live to the fullest.

Courage grows as we practice, gradually, increasing our abilities to achieve and maintain good self-care. Celebrating even small advances toward this goal will create a happier stance in which to live. Given time, empowerment is felt within one's self—and also within relationships. You too, can become encouraged to believe in your new abilities.

It is important to know every person has a right to carve out a good journey here on planet earth. There are many self-help books on library shelves. This workbook may be a beginning for some toward discovering how to "be the real me," one who has love for self and love for others, while working toward excellent relationships and is on track for finding soul's passion.

Write of an instance in the past wherein you now realize boundaries were needed, but didn't exist:____

(More space for writing)

How do you think that could have played out if set boundaries (with stated consequences) had been a part of the picture?___

It is important to have very real boundaries with yourself as it pertains to moving from addiction to recovery. Dealing with a repetitive desire to get high may feel pervasive at times. When the yearnings come, remember a quote by Dr. Barbara Krantz (who was once an addict). She spoke of answering drug addicts or alcoholics who ask, "Can I ever use substances in moderation?" She says, "No. Once your brain becomes a pickle, it can't go back to being a cucumber."[12]

A major boundary with self is involved for the sake of sobriety/recovery: With addiction, it is eminently important to stay on Medication-assisted-treatment (**MAT**).

---

[12]"Kluger, Jeffery. "Addiction By Doctor's Prescription." Special Time Edition, *The Science of Addiction What We Know. What We're Learning*," Meredith National Media Group, NY (2019), page 45.

On a scale of 1-10, how strong is your commitment to reach recovery through becoming substance free?   Enter that number, here:____

If you response is less than 10, do you intend to improve that number? Yes____   No____

If "no" is your response to that question, write the reason why below:____ (This will help you get clear with yourself)

Think of ways you could improve that number, if it is less than "10:___

Write of an instance during which reasonable boundaries were stated, yet not respected—and deliberately not allowed, within a relationship or a situation.___

Describe a current situation in which boundaries are needed within a personal relationship or situation.___

Write what *consequence* could be set in the event your boundaries are not respected and honored:___

As stated above, setting a consequence makes your boundary actual and effective.

For additional help, *Boundaries: When to Say Yes, How to Say No to Take Control of Your Life* offers excellent help with setting boundaries. *This* book authored by two psychotherapists, John Townsend and Henry Cloud is a superb and well-known resource. It offers immense assistance with assuring readers of their right to set boundaries, plus showing how to set and maintain them. A workbook, titled *Boundaries Workbook* by these two authors is also available and sure to compliment your efforts. (Both of these books are currently available on Amazon.com)

Explore your abilities

List here, abilities you are already aware of as being uniquely yours___

If you are inclined to deny having any specific abilities, this is something to discuss further with your counselor or friend. Most likely you are blocked from seeing your unique abilities, and your support team will help you identify these.

Plan toward further developing your unique abilities. Enter here what you would like your first step toward doing this to be___

The hope for this workbook is that it can help to empower you to reach a deep caring for yourself. Through this developed or renewed ability to value you, who you are and who you are not— you can move to higher realms of living. This growth will include paying attention to when you need to take time apart to evaluate pathways to good self-care, meaning what you can do to **find your center and to stay centered** during difficult times:

- when frustrated,
- when feeling down,
- when feeling highly stressed,
- when ashamed or angry at yourself.

This will call for honoring and identifying what you are feeling. Developing a practice of journaling daily helps stay on track with honesty. We are most integritous when we are at our center.

Rick Warren says, "It may be tough for you to read a message about integrity because you're replaying in your mind all the times you've fallen short, all the opportunities you had to show integrity but didn't, all the moral failures in your life. We could all make a similar list of failures. St. Augustine said that the confession of bad works is the beginning of good works. If you are serious about becoming a person of integrity, the first step is to admit that you haven't had integrity. You just admit that you don't always keep your promises. The first step [of one's self] in forgiveness is admitting your guilt . . . In this way you accept responsibility." Warren asks this question, "What's the best way to ensure that you are really accepting responsibility [addiction]? You're not going to like the answer, but you need to hear it anyway: The best way to get over your guilt is to tell one other person who loves you." [13] [14]

Warren is explaining a skill set of sharing your journey with a trusted person. This may be new for you. But, recovery will see you learning ways of being in the world. Learn all you can about healthy ways of living. Do your own research to assure personal integrity. Yet, **while using the Internet take care to use only trustworthy site sources**. A professor in one of my master's degree programs said, "There is a lot of horse muck on the Internet."

Two of my favorite sites while doing research related to health and mental health are the National Institute of Health at, **https://www.nih.gov/health-information** and SAMHSA at, **https://www.samhsa.gov/**

List here topics you want to research:__

---

[13] "Confess *your* trespasses to one another, and pray for one another, that you may be healed. The effective, fervent prayer of a righteous man avails much." (James 5:16).

[14] Warren, Rick, "How to Take the First Step to Integrity, https://pastorrick.com/how-to-take-the-first-step-to-integrity/ (Accessed February 13, 2020.)

More on managing stress

Think of this part of your journey as if you are taking up a new sport, like tennis or basketball. There will be many aspects of stress management that you will want to learn along with other specific skills for doing good self-care. Go for these! If you learn to manage stress you will find your journey to recovery much easier.

Knowledge is power. Consider the following National Institute of Health links for advancing your ability to handle stress well:

https://www.nimh.nih.gov/health/publications/stress/index.shtml

Use the Internet to learn how to avoid adrenaline rushes. Visit:

https://nccih.nih.gov/health/stress/relaxation.htm

Dr. Nora Volkow, director or the National Institute on Drug Abuse studies the neurological roots of addiction. She states, "Stress affects the way a person is able to anticipate the consequences of their actions. This happens because "the part of the prefrontal cortex that is involved in deliberative cognition is shut down by stress." This normally is helpful to a person, momentarily, yet as this expert points out, the frontal cortex is "even more inhibited in chronic substance users." Animal studies confirm stress can amplify a desire for drugs.[15]

Check out what SAMHSA has to offer while seeking recovery. Gaining all the information you can find on stress management will definitely help you succeed.

---

[15]Lemonick, Michael. The Science of Addiction. *Special Time Edition, the Science of Addiction What We Know. What We're Learning.* Book Excerpt: Meredith Corporation: NY (2019) p. 8.

You will have less stress if you can accept these three factors:

1) You are imperfect;

2) You are limited;

3) Recovery will take *as long as it takes*.

Grappling with these three factors may not appear to be a skill set but it truly is. These factors are ideally reckoned with throughout life. There is nothing here to be ashamed of. We are all in the same boat. You have abilities and gifts that I do not have. And, I have abilities and gifts that you do not have. Each of us is limited and all of us are imperfect. No one can do recovery perfectly.

What if I relapse

The truth is if relapse happens, it can serve to make you stronger and more knowledgeable. Yet, a relapse can bring a lot of shame. You may feel a load of guilt over relapsing, especially when you were doing very well prior to this. Hanging onto shame and guilt will only serve to *undermine who you are and what you are trying to do*. Let it go!

There may be fear that you "can't make it with recovery." Here is where you can look closely at what caused your relapse, becoming wiser going forward. An exercise titled, "Stop Thought" in the Addendum of this workbook (pages 84, alongside page 52) will help you learn how to recognize and release fear, disappointment, hurt and anger when these arise.

Avoiding relapses does take determination—but also **planning**. Emily Vona, Director of Arizona Treatment Center[16], says, "Relapse happens when people get complacent and put recovery too far down on the list of things they "need to do today." Planning and determination are equally important."

Stay on your Medication-assisted-treatment (**MAT**) as a solid way to recovery, purpose to trust God (or Higher Power) to help you day-by-day. Talk to God when you feel weak.

Consider praying daily for help in developing a true sense of your worth and stay true to truth, as you set your will to live sober in lasting recovery. You may choose prayer and "fasting" from substance abuse as a lifetime practice.

When you fear a relapse may happen, remember to call on God's help as many times during the day as you feel to do so. Scripture says, "Be still and know that I am God," (Psalms 46:10).

Prayer is 50% talking to God and 50% listening. Times of hearing God speak inwardly are blessed events. Learning to be still "in the

---

[16] For information on the Arizona Treatment Center, visit AZRecover.com

presence of the Most High" is a holy quest. It is all about holding silence within the softness of enjoying God, listening to hear what God may say. It is called "contemplation" for saints of the past and present. Very often silence is all that is heard, while you may wish to hear words. Yet, there is a message. Most likely saying something like, "Keep trusting. You are on a right track." We hear what our hearts can perceive.

The following quote from the National Institute of Health about recovery is included for reasons you will understand:

"Recovery from addiction, a chronic, relapse-prone disorder (Leshner, 1997), is a lifelong dynamic process. While we know a great deal about addiction, we know very little about recovery. The majority of studies conducted among substance abusers have follow-up periods ranging in length from 1 to 24 months - a short time relative to the lifelong challenges of recovery. What little is known about the natural history of addiction and recovery indicates that the recovery experience changes substantively over time and makes changing demands on the individual . . . "[17]

So, if relapse inadvertently takes place for you, see it as part of the learning process. Comfort yourself with knowing you have all it takes to strike a new beginning. One of the worse things you can do is to bad-mouth yourself, which will weaken rather than to strengthen you.

Think of it this way, if you drop your cell phone, do you pick it up and put it in your pocket, or do you stamp on it with your foot and grind it into the ground? Of course not. So be kind and caring toward yourself.

Apologize to yourself. Emily Vona, Director of the Arizona Treatment Center says, "Accept your own apology."

Let go the fear, each time it comes. Ask for help. Talk to your health provider about next steps.

---

[17] https://www.ncbi.nlm.nih.gov/pmc/articles/PMC1852519/ (Accessed January 29).

Relapses do not mean that you sink all the way to the bottom again. A onetime relapse does not have to turn into a month or a yearlong relapse. You have the ability to stop it from getting worse by bending your knee to it. Ask God to help you and to strengthen you. Ask yourself, "What happened, here? What brought on a relapse?" Write about this in the "Note Section" of this workbook. A note, made as you learn and progress, can greatly benefit you at points when you want to review them.

Prevention is key! Remember, that relapse after a period of recovery is statistically high for fatalities.

Being kind to yourself is a sign that you are learning to value who and what you are: a magnificent human being created to love and serve—in the progress of becoming. Mistakes are our greatest teachers. We learn what does not work. We go on.

It's not important how many times you have fallen. It is important how many times you have let God pick you up. You are still a remarkable person. God loves you. Listen to this! God loves you! His mercies are forever. Before you were even out of your mother's womb, He knew you would have to go through this within your learning experiences in this life. Now, trust. All you have to do is say "yes," I am going to trust. I am not alone, here. The best of all help has come alongside. *Love of self is a very large part of what God expects of us*: "You shall love the LORD[18] your God

---

[18] A brief explanation may help, here. Through the past 2000+ years it is the Lord who has been the refuge for many generations of people (perhaps totaling billions in number). We call ourselves "Christians," because of Christ and His teachings, which we attempt to follow. We do, of course, fail a lot, so please don't' be put off by the sinfulness you may have seen within one of us. This life is all about learning—learning to be who we truly hope to be. As Christians, we are working toward a powerful goal, one that is *to become like the Lord Jesus Christ*. Yet, individuals vary in their dedication. Clearly, even with the best of dedications, it will take an entire life time "on the path" to even partially achieve this. Please forgive us for the ways in which we fail to meet this magnificent goal within our lifetimes. Clearly, the nomenclature of "the Lord," was used in both the Old Testament, which was written by Hebrew prophets and scholars, as well as throughout the New Testament written by the first converts to Jesus Christ. It is easy to see, through this that both Jews and Christians put their trust in and serve the same Lord God of heaven.

with all your heart, with all your soul, with all your strength, and with all your mind, and your neighbor as yourself" (Luke 10:27).

Once you have Medication-assisted treatment **(MAT)** on-board you will be wiser. You will know what you need to do differently.

Work concertedly on gaining some new coping skills, which will help you put your life back together. This will then bring the great pleasure of paying your own way in life and will majorly help you succeed in reaching recovery. You may need to live pretty skinny in order to get your life back on course. The practice of self-denial will help you as you discern this truth: There is something at work in your soul, calling you to a deep and meaningful journey. There is more of God's goodness inside of you than you can recognize.

Meanwhile, going without non-essentials will help develop the impetus to see the value of self-denial and embrace it.

Avoiding relapse means you are growing—coming into a love of self and others. Celebrate and thank God for every moment you are saying "NO" to all felt urgings towards relapsing. It is important to consider helping your body recover by abiding by the best possible health practices: eating nourishing food, getting 8 hours of sleep each night, drink plenty of water and let people love on you. Take the hugs. Receive any "good words" or compliments they offer you. It is one thing to hear them, but quite another to take the words in . . . truly receiving them, allowing good feelings to nurture your soul.

Place distance between yourself and your addiction. You are NOT the addiction and the addiction is not you.

Without a doubt, addiction and substance abuse are a major problem in the US. A survey conducted by the Substance Abuse and Mental Health Services Administration found that as many as 90 percent of people who most need drug rehab do not receive it. Once a person is on-board, receiving medical help for the purpose of recovery, gratitude can become a powerful aid in recovery. Gratitude expressed often for having medication available, which is mostly paid by insurance or State programs, is a factor that is likely to be a mighty force of empowerment to people who are intending to stay sober. Studies in a medical field called "psychoneuroimmunology" or PNI, have proven what goes on in the psyche affects nearly every system in the body. Gratitude—being thankful—changes the body's chemistry and brings on endorphin flows. A quote from Summer Allen may well put you on course for living a life of ubiquitous gratitude: "After 15 years of research, we know that **gratitude** is a key to psychological well-being. Gratitude can make people happier, improve their relationships, and potentially **even** counter-act **depression** and **suicidal thoughts**.[19]

[19]   https://greatergood.berkeley.edu/article/item/is_gratitude_good_for_your_health (Accessed April 30, 2020.)

Finding the Divine

Whether we realize it or not, spirituality is the centrality of all human beings. We all have "spirit." What a person believes about spirituality is important to identify, regardless of what our beliefs are about what "spirit" is, or is not—it will indeed be central in life. It is the spirit of a person through which empowerment arises.

This workbook will not present information about world religions. The Constitution of the USA supports the dignity and right of each person to choose what they will believe to be true about life and how it should be lived, also about death and eternity.

As an author, with degrees in both psychology and theology, I extend, here, what I consider to be the best of all beliefs for readers who seek to "find the Divine" within their journey here on earth. Based on all my studies, I believe the Bible contains more psychology (and the best of it) than all the books of my library.

It is where theology lies par excellence. But, please know that the gist of what this workbook covers are the tools for getting past addictions—and will work well for you—no matter what your spiritual beliefs. My intent is for this work to carefully respect the beliefs of all while being majorly helpful in the struggle against addictions.

In the Addendum of this workbook, I include two pages titled, "Biblical passages that soothe the soul" which readers can turn to at any point when emotional pain is felt. During my 7+ decades of life, these words have held tremendous power to assure, satisfy and fortify my soul. Based on that, I know an even greater amount of empowerment will come to readers if prayer and the helps billions of people continue to find in Scripture are a part of the work. (See page 96, in the Addendum, titled, "About the Bible – why read it?" And, see page 99, "Biblical passages that soothe the soul.")

For those of you who have already experienced God helping you in your life, you know there is a mighty Power beyond yourself.

By including this "Power" in your sincere recovery work will provide opportunity to more quickly and surely achieve your goals.

Assurance of forgiveness

Throughout the Bible God inspires us to believe all mistakes—all sins—are forgiven, erased from our pasts once we repent of them. Repentance sees us turning away from behaviors that were harmful to ourselves and others.

The Scripture passages listed below offer helps for letting go of past mistakes and failures. These passages will grant assurance for applying forgiveness on a daily basis. Only the Bible, known to believers as "the Word of God," can make it possible to accept the truth of this freedom from the past. You may want to refer periodically to these four Biblical passages that assure us of the truth that God grants forgiven when we ask for it:

Isaiah 1:18
"Come now, and let us reason together," Says the LORD, "Though your sins are like scarlet they shall be as white as snow; though they are red like crimson, they shall be as wool."

Psalms 103: 12-14
"As far as the east is from the west, so far has He removed our transgressions. As a father pities his children, so the LORD pities those who fear Him. For He knows our frame; He remembers that we are dust."

John 3:16
"For God so loved the world that he gave his one and only Son, that whoever believes in him shall not perish but have eternal life."

Romans 10:9-10
". . . That if you confess with your mouth the Lord Jesus and believe in your heart that God has raised Him from the dead, you will be saved. For with the heart one believes unto righteousness, and with the mouth confession is made unto salvation."

Daily reading of Scripture is what keeps me on track with my efforts to truly let go the past and live solidly in the present.

Medical research discovery: the physical and spiritual come together for transcendence

It does seem clear that one's use of alcohol or opioids may allow a "momentary" sense of "transcending" the pressures, confusions, frustrations, disappointments, stressor and griefs of life. Trouble comes when once these are used long enough (or for some immediately upon first trying them), the person gets "hooked." This is often a catastrophe of "evilish" dimensions. Now, like many others, you may suffer major struggles as life has taken a disastrous spin.

If you are not already on medication assisted treatment, please seek a health provider and get that care immediately.

In addition, it has now been scientifically proven that the human brain itself has specific abilities to help us transcend. Transcendence is a place where one's spirit is elevated above all else that is happening in life. There is a sense of joy and peace—with an indescribable calmness.

An explanation of this truth can be found in *Why God Won't Go Away - Brain Science & the Biology of* Belief by Andrew Newberg, M.D., Eugene D'Aquili, M.D., and Vince Rause.[20] These medical scientists write of how exciting it was for them to discover what takes place in the brain when people pray or meditate. Their research involved creating SPECT MRI brain images of people while they were praying or meditating.

These doctors did their research, without regard for any religious beliefs or practices of their own. Through this work they discovered how the brain is built for transcendence. Their remarkable research brought attention to the very location within the human brain where this takes place as it is clearly identifiable, consistently lighting up when prayer or meditation is

---

[20] Newberg, Andrew. D'Aquili, Eugene. and Rause, Vince. *Why God Won't Go Away – Brain Science & the Biology of Belief*. (New York: Ballantine Books, 2002).

entered and continued for 12 or more minutes. Their research identified the where and when of mystical states as these take place for us as humans. These are experienced, of course, to varying intensities.

As detailed in their book, the researchers scientifically prove that our brains are tailor-made for linking up with and entering the empowering presence of our Creator. We have the ability to elicit this place of wholeness through meditation and prayer. It is now proven that our brains can bring us into an amazing transcendence.

Experiment with the above: Set a timer for 12 minutes. Turn your phone off and quiet your mind. Let all thoughts slide off the screen of your mind as they arise. And, they will. When thoughts of the work you need to get done break in, gently bring your mind back into prayer or quietude. Repeating a phrase of your choice can help you stay centered. It can also be useful to identify a word or phrase to speak when thoughts try to interrupt, like, "I am safe," "peace," "rest," "at home." Choose what seems most helpful to you. Even a longer sentence can be use, something like, "I greatly appreciate the gift of life."

Just settle and sink sweetly into this place where all is entrusted into the Creator's care. Notice what you feel. Or, perhaps it can take a number of trial runs before you find that place of transcendence of your soul…the "uplift." Make this a practice that is ideally combined with reading Scriptural passages before or after your time of shutting all down in quietude in order to enter into and accept the stillness with God.[21]

For a blessed, quieting music experience, visit:
https://www.youtube.com/watch?v=FKWGSzxtcZA

Truth be known, both prayer and reading of Scripture passages can bring us into astounding realms of reality with God. These doctors mentioned above became exceedingly excited in learning

---

[21] "Be still, and know that I *am* God;
I will be exalted among the nations,
I will be exalted in the earth!" (Psalm 46:10).

we are created to experience transcendence wherein the soul is at a place of rest and assurance that life is good.

Perhaps this is what Scripture refers to as "the secret place of the Most High."[22]

My personal experience with prayer and meditation is that peace, contentment and joy are interwoven when my heart and mind are at rest. A gentle uplifting of one's being takes place. Transcendence! I feel loved and united with God during such prayer times. This is not a time wherein I am asking for anything for myself. I am just setting all aside except to be with God. I feel sure there is a "joining," here, where love encounters love—resulting in a grand reward for body, soul and spirit.

Through this we can transcend all the pain of life. It just takes the practice of "entering in."

Mike Cardello, our local Celebrate Recovery director, says, "Find God on your own ground. Challenge Him—for you to know He is *real*! The love of other believers showed me who Christ is. For a time, I needed someone else's faith until I found my own." Mike has a story of recovery that brought tears to my eyes.

Along with the support of your accountability team, counseling will accentuate the cognitive behavioral aspect of this workbook. Counseling supports a process through which you will become more able to reach the underlying issues of your past, opening the door to the discovery of a new future wherein you can truly be the person you want to be.

Through 24 years of work as a mental health counselor and clinical Board certified chaplain, I have witnessed renewed lives. People are healed most expediently and most lastingly through the practice of ancient habits: prayer, study, worship and service. It is called "The Way" in Scripture. This way of living will see you

---

[22] "He who dwells in the secret place of the Most High shall abide under the shadow of the Almighty." (Psalm 91:1, NKJ)."

Cycling through five spiritual practices of learning, turning, praying, worshiping and blessing the lives of others. This "Way" of living a loving life starts with learning to truly love God, but also to truly love yourself. This will empower you to "rest"—rest from your anxieties, your fears, your frustrations, resentments, disappointments . . . letting go the angst of life so peace, love and joy can fill your heart and bring the glory of living to your soul.

When you are in counseling, a place where you know confidentiality is the rule, your heart can speak. And, as it does—you hear yourself. You begin to put it together so to speak. You know more clearly what is hurting, what you are doing to hurt yourself, what you want most to happen. With the acceptance and support of this other listening person, feel joined. You come to respect yourself more fully and to respect what you want to happen henceforth.

The best tool I have within my counseling practice (meaning what people are most often thankful for) is to always include God as I work with individuals. I discover what their understanding is of God (or Higher Power). Their intake paperwork includes a release to sign, assuring them that "God will be part of this work." Even atheists have signed that agreement and have done well within my practice. What I know is that God takes us just as we are. I always want to introduce people to Christ. Sometimes that happens and sometimes it does not. Both in this workbook and in counseling I respect where people are most comfortable with this very important fulcrum of life.

Christian beliefs are extended here along with some scriptural passages, to further enrich and empower readers, *in the event you are open to considering them*.

If this part of the workbook is not what you find comfort in believing, then please do one of two things:

1) Give it a read, maybe even try it on for size, as you may very well find it to be amazingly wondrous, such as trillions of

people (among the living and the dead) have since the beginning of time; or:

2) **Please just move past this portion of the workbook.**
Continue to page 81, which will link you up with more tools for reaching recovery.

None of us can do life perfectly—nor is there a "perfect recovery."

In the path Jesus called "the way," Christians know we can only accept the covering of the perfection of Jesus Christ who supplied that to us through His death on the cross, followed by His resurrection. Deciding to be His follower means we take on *His perfection*. How can this be? The December, 2019, issue of Christianity Today says it well, based a Biblical passage in 2 Cor. 5:21), "Just as God looks upon the Lord Christ as sin (because our sins were reckoned to him), so He sees the sinner as just and completely perfect." God gives to the sinner a gift—totally undeserved: "the innocence and righteousness of Christ." [23]
It is like we wear a robe of Christ's perfection that covers our every sin—our every imperfection—based on our trust in what He has done for us. God's kingdom within the world is comprised of "righteousness, peace and joy in the Holy Spirit" (Romans 14:17). It is different from "the world" we see—work, play and ponder in. It is a kingdom that we, as people, *choose* as a state of being for our souls.

Dr. Gerald G. May understood this well when he wrote, "Addiction cannot be defeated by the human will acting on its own, nor by the human will opting out and turning everything over to divine will. Instead, the power of grace flows most fully when human will chooses to act in harmony with divine will. In practical terms, this means staying in a situation, being willing to confront it as it is, remaining responsible for the choices one makes in response to it, but at the same time turning to God's grace, protection, and guidance as the ground for one's choices and behavior. It is the difference between testing God by avoiding one's own

[23]Christianity Today, https://www.christianitytoday.com/history/issues/issue-10/from-archives-on-christian-perfection.html (Accessed February 3, 2020).

responsibilities and trusting God as one acts responsibly. Responsible human freedom becomes authentic spiritual surrender, and authentic spiritual surrender is nothing other than responsible human freedom. Here, in the condition of humble dignity, the power of addiction can be overcome."[24]

The above words of Dr. May involve an adventure of body, mind and spirit. Truly remarkable occurrences—even astounding happenstances—can take place when you choose this state of being for your soul on a regular basis. Herein lies an adventure and it involves God.

---

[24] May, Gerald. *Addiction and Grace: Love and Spirituality in Healing Addictions.* (New York: HarpOne, 1998.) p. 136.

FDA announces more good news!

The FDA is taking new steps to advance the development of improved treatments for opioid use disorder and to make sure these medicines are accessible to the patients who need them. "That includes promoting the development of better drugs, and also facilitating market entry of generic versions of approved drugs to help ensure broader access," said FDA Commissioner Scott Gottlieb, MD, in a press release.[25]

The FDA is also taking "new steps" to address the unfortunate stigma that is often associated with the use of opioid replacement therapy as a means to successfully treat addiction.

A common false belief is that patients addicted to opioids, who are transitioned onto medicines like buprenorphine, are swapping one addiction for another. This is not true. These are people who have regained control of their lives and have ended the destructive outcomes that result from being addicted to opioids. When coupled with other social, medical, and psychological services, medication-assisted treatment is proving to be an effective approach for opioid dependence.[26]

Medication-assisted-treatment **(MAT)** is provided for alcohol addiction as well as opioid addiction. Several medications are used within MAT, which superbly address the cravings and withdrawal symptoms for both of these addictions.[27]

The vast reality of widespread opioid addiction in the US begs for attention. More than 2 million Americans abuse opioids and more than 90 Americans die by opioid overdose every day.[28] Going

---

[25] https://www.fda.gov/news-events/press-announcements/statement-fda-commissioner-scott-gottlieb-md-fdas-new-steps-modernize-drug-development-improve. (Accessed June 27, 2020.)

[26] https://www.fda.gov/news-events/press-announcements/fda-approves-first-generic-versions-suboxone-sublingual-film-which-may-increase-access-treatment. (Accessed June 27, 2020.)

[27] **https://www.samhsa.gov/medication-assisted-treatment/treatment/naltrexone**.(Accessed June 27, 2020.)

[28] https://www.asahq.org/whensecondscount/pain-management/opioid-treatment/opioid-abuse/ (Accessed June 10, 2020.)

forward, the good news of carrying hope needs to lie solidly alongside what continues to be a startling challenge. The opioid reality shouts, "More must be done!

Medication-assisted treatment (MAT) cuts a person's "risk of death from all causes in half."[29] Sadly, as many as 90 percent of people who need drug rehab do not receive it.[30]

This workbook is prepared to encourage people to do all possible to live a normal life without addictions. There are effective medications available, suited to facilitate sobriety. Recovery medication (MAT) is most effective when counselling and therapy are included. Counselling and other behavioral therapies are essential for SUD patients. Behavioral experts can help target the underlying reason(s) for opioid use. Efforts to determine what "triggers you" can be taken, along with steps for finding ways to cope with the pain and stress of life. These, among other helps professionals are able to give, are imminently important steps for reaching and maintaining recovery.

As you finish this workbook, if you have not yet asked your health provider for information on Medication-assisted treatment **(MAT)**, please do so. This is vitally important.

Treating addiction with medication can greatly change the effects of drug addiction, *allowing a* person *to work and live a normal life*. MAT is saving lives. To find MAT health providers in your area, enter your zip code in the locator at this website: **https://findtreatment.gov/**

Please use the **annotated Bibliography provided on page 110**, as the best and most updated information on treatment options. Advanced research pertaining to opioid addiction are mostly found online.

---

[29] "FDA Approves First Generic Versions of Suboxone Sublingual Film," **https://www.managedcaremag.com/news/20180619/fda-approves-first-generic-versions-suboxone-sublingual-film.** (Accessed October 19, 2019.)

---

[30] **https://americanaddictioncenters**.org/rehab-guide/success-rates-and-statistics (Acccessed June 27, 2020.)

Addendum

**Please enjoy the following aids for
Strengthening your skills and
spiritual growth.**

"Stop thought!" technique

As you monitor your thoughts, make sure you don't allow the dark or negative ones that raise unfair criticism of yourself.

Remember: Feelings follow thoughts. The feelings we experience come from what our thoughts are presenting to us. Even with the exceptions (when feelings arise from something we see or hear, or with a flash back memory) the technique below has proven to work for many.

Some thoughts become very persistent. Many people have found the following technique to work effectively. Here is how to stop difficult, persistent thoughts when they come:

Think or say, "Stop thought!" (Conceptualize)

Mentally visualize each letter – slowly spell it out:

S T O P T H O U G H T

The thought can return. Simply repeat, "Stop thought!"
 (Train your brain.)

The thought may persist. Work the mind, "Stop thought!"

Do this repetitively. The thought will stop when you continue repeating your command, "Stop thought!" If you are alone, at the time, say, "Stop thought!" out loud. Otherwise, it still works when you say, "Stop thought!" quietly within.

This technique has also worked for people during sleep when thoughts arise keeping them awake.

My Child . . .

You may not know me, but I know everything about you.
Psalm 139:1

I know when you sit down and when you rise up
Psalm 139:2

I am familiar with all your ways.
Psalm 139:3

Even the very hairs on your head are numbered.
Matthew 10:29-31

For you were made in my image.
Genesis 1:27

In me you live and move and have your being.
Acts 17:28

For you are my offspring.
Acts 17:28

I knew you even before you were conceived.
Jeremiah 1:4-5

I chose you when I planned creation.
Ephesians 1:11-12

You were not a mistake, for all your days are written in my book.
Psalm 139:15-16

I determined the exact time of your birth and where you would live.
Acts 17:26

You are fearfully and wonderfully made.
Psalm 139:14

I knit you together in your mother's womb.
Psalm 139:13

And brought you forth on the day you were born.
Psalm 71:6

I have been misrepresented by those who don't know me.
John 8:41-44

I am not distant and angry, but am the complete expression of love
1st John 4:16

And it is my desire to lavish my love on you,
1st John 3:1

Simply because you are my child and I am your Father.
1st John 3:1

I offer you more than your earthly father ever could,
Matthew 7:11

For I am the perfect father.
Matthew 5:48

Every good gift that you receive comes from my hand,
James 1:17

For I am your provider and I meet all your needs.
Matthew 6:31-33

My plan for your future has always been filled with hope.
Jeremiah 29:11

Because I love you with an everlasting love.
Jeremiah 31:3

My thoughts toward you are countless as the sand on the seashore
Psalm 139:17-18

and I rejoice over you with singing.
Zephaniah 3:17

I will never stop doing good to you,
Jeremiah 32:40

For you are my treasured possession.
Exodus 19:5

I desire to establish you with all my heart and all my soul
Jeremiah 32:41

And I want to show you great and marvelous things.
Jeremiah 33:3

If you seek me with all your heart, you will find me.
Deuteronomy 4:29

Delight in me and I will give you the desires of your heart.
Psalm 37:4

For it is I who gave you those desires.
Philippians 2:13

I am able to do more for you than you could possibly imagine.
Ephesians 3:20

For I am your greatest encourager.
2nd Thessalonians 2:16-17

Also I am the Father who comforts you in all your troubles.
2nd Corinthians 1:3-4

When you are brokenhearted, I am close to you.
Psalm 34:18

As a shepherd carries a lamb, I have carried you close to my heart.
Isaiah 40:11

One day I will wipe away every tear from your eyes.
Revelation 21:3-4

And I'll take away all the pain you have suffered on this earth.
Revelation 21:3-4

I am your Father, and I love you even as I love my son, Jesus.
John 17:23

For in Jesus, my love for you is revealed.
John 17:26

He is the exact representation of my being.
Hebrews 1:3

He came to demonstrate that I am for you, not against you.
Romans 8:31

And to tell you that I am not counting your sins.
2nd Corinthians 5:18-19

Jesus died so that you and I could be reconciled.
2nd Corinthians 5:18-19

His death was the ultimate expression of my love for you.
1st John 4:10

I gave up everything I loved that I might gain your love.
Romans 8:31-32

If you receive the gift of my son, Jesus, you receive me,
1st John 2:23

And nothing will ever separate you from my love again.
Romans 8:38-39

Come home and I'll throw the biggest party heaven has ever seen!
Luke 15:7

I have always been Father, and will always be Father.
Ephesians 3:14-15

My question is . . . Will you be my child?
John 1:12-13

I am waiting for you.
Luke 15:11-32

Love, Your Dad, Almighty God

LIFE – what is it all about?

Now for further pondering of the "why" question at the beginning of this segment of the workbook:

One day while working as a chaplain, I was asked one of the hardest of all questions, "What is this life all about?" The patient added, "My Company took a tumble, my wife lost her job and I was diagnosed yesterday with a terminal condition. I've tried to stay on top financially . . . I've tried to lose all this weight. How can I believe in a God who allows such misery?"

I inwardly thought, "You place a lot of trust, expecting me to answer that question. I did the best I could while at his bedside as a comforter. Yet, felt surely it was not enough. Now, at home, I reflect on my response.

We are created to be in relationship with the Creator. God wanted children. In the first book of the Bible, we see how that turned out. Not well--because God built free will into our package. We get to choose whether to believe and live by some rules (so justice can exist on planet earth), or, we follow and live by whatever *we think or feel* we want at any given moment. The Bible reveals how it goes for people who honor God with their lives by putting their trust in Him and enjoying a vital relationship. It also shows how tragically things go for those who do only *as they please* giving little thought to consequences.

Many of us start learning at that point—learning how to engage with our Creator. Scripture calls it "sup"[31] which means we commune with Him. Supping forms relationship. It is for sure a love relationship. We learn to seek God's guidance through prayer and savoring the scriptures which is called His Word. Here is where a phenomenal relationship begins. Words cannot describe the joys of it. Love is the most powerful entity in the universe. I speak of heartfelt, unselfish love—extended as valued as equals. We hold potential of growing to be more and more like God . . .

---

[31] Revelation 3:20, "Behold, I stand at the door and knock. If anyone hears My voice and opens the door, I will come in to him and dine with him, and he with Me."

whose love is unconditionally.

Scripture tells us, "God is love." Scripture also says if we claim to love Him yet cannot love others we are liars. Wow. That can be scary.

1 John 4:7 makes it plain, "Beloved, let us love one another, for love is of God; and everyone who loves is born of God and knows God. [8] He who does not love does not know God, for God is love. It seems most likely that love is the greatest power in the universe—and that *the more we love* the more we become like our Creator.

The opposite is true, as we can be selfishly grasping for what we want in life, with little thought of others. We can even be outright mean, thinking nothing of stealing from others and even taking their lives before their time is up.

Looking at history it is easy to see there is plenty of temptation to walk away from God's love—that is until we open our human hearts to Him. Then, slowly there is a stream of tender care that can grow deep and wide. It is God's love pouring through us as we invest ourselves in the best kinds of causes, especially those providing safety, health, healing and equality.

This earth can be a little bit of heaven on earth, or it can be a little bit of hell. In the latter case, we have the human race causing much to regret. On the former, there are a lot of us who take love to be our primary cause for our being given this great journey of life.

It does seem this globe is a fitting place for souls to be tried. We get to choose which side of things we want to be on. If God had not built free will into each human heart, we would simply live as a bunch of puppets.

To be sure, in this journey, here on the globe, we all enter the master of all "universities." We are on task for learning—learning from our mistakes and also from our successes. Our mistakes can be our best teachers, yet so often these become the most painful. It hurts very much to see ourselves falling short, and then having to backtrack as we step onto the right path, again. It is humbling, but there is healing.

We have this lifetime, with many explorations of choosing "the right" and "the wrong," in order to gain the wisdom that fires the soul and sees us denying ourselves so as to live toward what is best for all. A path that blesses is one in which we lean into the experience of making it easier for others, especially the ones who are suffering without having done anything to bring it on for themselves: People who are mentally ill, those who are developmentally challenged, people who have been accidentally or criminally maimed and those who find themselves enslaved by addictions.

Only God knows the circumstance of another, such as the man in the hospital bed who posed one of the hardest of all questions. What I had to give him was a compassionate presence and a "word" of encouragement.

So, it is about giving our all, while experiencing felt limitation. Surely, the dream portrays Christ simply being able to stand as a loving, listening presence as the person suffered. That's also where we are as humans in ministry to others.

I got the point. Perhaps we do a harder thing? How much easier if only the miraculous touch of Christ was ours to extend.

Who doesn't long for the miraculous power to heal, above and beyond the experience of simply being prayerful and encouraging? Yet, we forge on in faith. Truth be known, chaplaincy has seen me grow. I have come to believe that being my little, mostly helpless presence in common, ordinary ways of faith is more powerful than I will ever perceive. I represent the Father—the Creator—while there at the bedside.

My call is to trust He will take over as I leave. Here is the blessing I carry away . . . and it is a blessing that sees me keep coming back. The miracle is my obedience . . . to keep on loving, keep going to the bedsides ministering love.

**"And we are put on earth a little space
That we might learn to bear the beams of love."**

William Blake

Tears: How they help the body heal as well as the soul

By Joy Le Page Smith (copied from www.healing-with-Joy.com)

Healing the soul is like peeling an onion. The layers of pain, resentment, bitterness, and sorrow come off one by one. No matter how many conferences attended and books read in hopes of getting more comfortable in our skins, most of us come to a notable realization: The hidden pain in our psyches hasn't gone away. It takes more than understanding. We are going to have to deal with it.

Here is the crux of the matter: If we want to be whole, we have to fight against all inclinations to gulp down feelings. Instead, when we feel tears at the corners of our eyes, we just *admit* what we are feeling, then *allow* the tears to flow, in a place where we feel safe. Most often, this takes place in privacy. Without a doubt, your body and your soul are healthier when you let those tears flow. Trust this natural, God-given process. Remind yourself that this emotional work does pay off. Freedom from your inner pain is on the way. Days of living with less stress lie ahead. Learning to grieve life's losses in this manner was a major factor in my becoming well after having to wage a serious battle to stay alive.

My "Get Well Program" involved praying, meditating, and studying Scriptures. However, I also journaled and listened to my dreams. One dream in particular spoke loud and clear about all my inner angst. In this dream, I am shown a huge mountain of frozen tears. The dream scene is an awesomely cold place! I awaken knowing that a piece of truth has paid me a visit. I see, clearly, that a mountain of frozen tears resides within my psyche. Those frozen tears need to come down, but they have to come down slowly, not all at once. I have to own up to all that stored grief, now so remote and hard to reach.

Eventually, my mountain of frozen tears began to thaw, allowing me to feel and to release that old, buried pain. I learned the value of tears and the need to let them have their way when they want to come. Jesus said, "You will know the truth and the truth will set you free" (John 8:32). The fact remains that *coming to truth* can take a lot of time and diligent effort when we have repressed a great deal of emotion, hoping it will "go away"--if we just stay busy enough. Or, drink enough … do enough drugs … recreate more. Clearly, if we want the change which brings a better life--one that is honoring to God--we have to do the work. And, for a lot of us, tears are part of it.

The truth about tears is that they help to heal our psyche (soul). And, amazingly enough, this little bit of water that begs to run down our faces *helps our bodies*.

Science indicates that tears are always present in the eyes and contain water, mucins, proteins, oils and electrolytes to keep the eyes moist, protect the eyes and facilitate the smooth movement of the lids over the surface. Tears are essential and their functions are many.

William H. Frey II, Ph.D. and Muriel Langseth, are authors of *Crying: The Mystery of Tears.*[1] Dr. Frey, a neuroscientist, at the Regions Hospital in St. Paul, Minnesota, suggests that physical benefits are gained through releasing emotional tears. He studied tears for 15 years, analyzing two types: 1) tears that come while crying when we are emotionally upset or stressed; and 2) tears arising from eye irritants, including onions. Dr. Frey and his colleagues also found that all tears are not the same and that stress-induced tears have a 24% higher protein concentration than tears caused by eye irritants. Dr. Frey proposed that weeping is an excretory process which facilitates the removal of substances that build up during times of emotional stress.[32]

One of the compounds found by Dr. Frey and his colleagues in human tears is Adrenocorticotropic Hormone (ACTH). This chemical is known to increase in the blood during stress. Dr. Frey's studies demonstrate that 85% of women and 73% of men

---

[32] Frey, William, Langseth, Muriel, *The Mystery of Tears* (Minneapolis: Winston Press, 1977).

feel better after crying. This indicates that suppressing tears over long periods of time may reduce our ability to alleviate stress, while increasing our risk of stress-related disorders, which include high blood pressure, heart problems, certain ulcers, and perhaps even memory loss.

More and newer research is showing that our bodies are helped when we pay attention to those moments when we feel tears arising, or when we have a lump in the throat. On an Internet site, Nurse Connect, in a posting titled "Nursing Dynamics and Clinical Issues," a nurse writes: "Without tears most nurses would be emotional wrecks. Let's face it, nursing is an emotional profession; on any given day we may witness pain, suffering and death, or extreme joy, relief and gratitude … encouraging a colleague not to cry, to 'be strong,' is detrimental to their psyche." This nurse concluded that chemicals built up in the body during stressful moments are removed by tears. We all have challenges, disappointments, and stressful times. Yielding to a good cry is a definite way of lowering our stress level and potentially helping our bodies to release harmful stress-related chemicals.

Ultimately, allowing our tears, permits both physical and emotional benefits. For one, tears carry a promise for better times ahead. We can be certain that clarity about what is at the root of our sadness, confusion or anxiety brings a certain joy of its own. Progress is gained and we are encouraged to keep moving forward with increased understanding about how to help our bodies stay healthy.

About the Bible – why read it?

Many people have not read the Bible. Reasons vary, but recently one man put it this way, "It is hard to put it all together and glean what I am meant to understand." Since reading the entire Bible once a year for at least a decade, I see God throughout as being for us—not at all against us—wanting us to be blessed. He has definite mercy, acceptance and forgiveness to offer us. The overall picture is that God allows us freedom to choose, learn and grow while enjoying divine guidance. When we get out of line, meaning we do something that is not loving and kind, we get a little nudge from our consciences. So, God is all about helping us live in a life that brings joy and stability. God is always available to help us.

In the Old Testament God was at work, forming a people who would honor him. But, historically the Israelite nation, initiated as "God's people," perpetually went their own way. (The pattern of humanity, common to us all.) God's plan was to bring the Messiah to the world through them, so He had strict rules, wanting the Israelites to follow His ways versus their own ways. That was a struggle for all involved, until the Savior of the world came through Christ. Now, God's plan became open to all people who put their trust in Him. To help people who are interested in knowing more about what Scriptures offer, I am listing below a number of passages that hold power to give hope, extend truth and heal one's heart. Applying these Scriptures to life will immensely help your recovery process.

The Bible helps us reach a right relationship with God by showing His acceptance, love and mercy towards us. The Bible shows us how God sees our every need and loves us intensely.
Below is a sampling of Scripture passages for those who would like a limited glimpse of what the Bible is indicating.

Every Scripture included in this workbook is extended for the purpose of bringing healing to your mind, body, and spirit. Reading the Bible and asking God to heal you grants the power needed to follow your heart while using the greatest wisdom of all ages. This is the very thing that will help you get free of dependence on substances that dump you in what is perhaps the darkest of all pits . . . or even rob you of time here on earth.

Since this workbook is created for people struggling with addictions, the following four passages address how God helps us out of "the pit" where each of us find ourselves at points in life:

Lamentations 3:55

 I called on Your name, O Lord, from the lowest pit. You have heard my voice: "Do not hide Your ear from my sighing, from my cry for help."

Job 33:28

"He has redeemed my soul from going to the pit, and my life shall see the light."

Psalm 103:4

"Who redeems your life from the pit, who crowns you with lovingkindness and compassion;"

Psalm 40:2

"He brought me up out of the pit of destruction, out of the miry clay, and He set my feet upon a rock making my footsteps firm."

Four scriptures that assure us of our being forgiven:

Daniel 9:9

"The Lord our God is merciful and forgiving, even though we have rebelled against him . . ."

Psalm 103:12

"As far as the east is from the west, so far has he removed our transgressions from us."

Micah 7:18-19[b]

"You will again have compassion on us; you will tread our sins underfoot and hurl all our iniquities into the depths of the sea."

Colossians. 3:13

"Bear with each other and forgive one another if any of you has a grievance against someone. Forgive as the Lord forgave you."

Knowing we have been forgiven creates an obligation on our parts to forgive those people who have harmed us. Forgiveness is a process. It takes as long as it takes to keep setting the will to forgive. It isn't easy, but entirely possible with God's help.

Biblical passages that soothe the soul

Isaiah 30:15, "For thus says the Lord GOD, the Holy One of Israel: In returning and rest you shall be saved; in quietness and confidence shall be your strength. But you would not . . . ."

Isaiah 26:3- "You will keep *him* in perfect peace,
whose mind *is* stayed *on You,* because he trusts in You."

In Revelations 3:20, Jesus Christ speaks, "Behold, I stand at the door and knock. If anyone hears My voice and opens the door, I will come in to him and dine with him, and he with Me."

Salvation comes to the soul through simply saying "yes" to that "knock," which is the call of Christ to enter your heart, your life.

A simple prayer is added here in the event you are ready to ask Jesus Christ to "come in and be Lord of your life." For sure, prayer is about speaking to God in words that come natural for you. Revise the following, if you wish. It is all about what YOU want to say to the the Lord. In case it is helpful, here is a possible prayer to use:

"Lord Jesus Christ, I have heard the knock on my heart's door. *I accept your call to enter my life.* I confess my sins and ask for your forgiveness. *I acknowledge You as my Savior and I am* asking You to enter my life. I pray to be guided by Your Holy Spirit from now on. I may have failures, but I am now seeking to be a 'new creature' in You. Amen."

Stop to savor your heart's felt release here.

An additional prayer to use at any time when it feels helpful:

"Lord, I believe you can strengthen me to the point where You can use my life—gifts and my talents in the service of your kingdom. <u>Your kingdom come, Your will be done</u>. I am Yours . . . for I surrender my soul to you, Lord Jesus Christ. Amen."

Always know that "prayer" is anything you want to say to the Lord—in your own words.

Write the date for saying this prayer, as this is your spiritual birthday! _____

It will be a delight if you go to my website and tell me about it at www.healing-with-Joy.com

Celebrate this occasion

You are now "reborn" – born of the Spirit of God! It is appropriate even to rejoice.

Nehemiah 8:10, "…The joy of the Lord is your strength." Please note that when people do choose to accept Jesus Christ as Lord and Savior, it is common to feel unworthy due to mistakes of the past. Yet, all that is needed is to ask for these marks in the heart, called sins, to be made clean. From that point on the precious Presence of God awakens and enlivens your spirit. Once you have repented and have accepted Jesus as your Lord and Savior, you can know without a doubt that you are forgiven.

For defeating shame over past mistakes and bad decisions, here is the promise to go back to each time it is needed, "*There is* therefore now no condemnation to those who are in Christ Jesus, who do not walk according to the flesh, but according to the Spirit," (Romans 8:1).

After a decision to ask Christ to abide with us, and to guide us, life does change. And certainly, we are never alone again. Scripture carries many amazing statements. Ponder this from 2 Corinthians 4:7," . . . we have this treasure in earthen vessels that the Excellency of the power may be of God, and not of us."

Gradually life is changed. And certainly, we are never alone again. God is as near as our breath—in fact, He abides in our breath! This call definitely empowers you as you call on God at every moment you feel weak, needing help, or just want to "feel the connection."

Here is a verse of Scripture that I use at times of temptation or when I fear harm: Proverbs 18:10, "The name of the LORD *is* a strong tower; the righteous run to it and are safe."

Welcome to the family of God that recognizes the Holy Spirit of Jesus Christ indwells the heart and soul of believers!

<u>The first thing to do</u> as a new Christian: Find other Christians who understand your decision for Christ. They will help you grow in your Christian faith. Going to church will give you a family within this chosen walk with God. Here, you will experience worshiping God within community.

Show up in the clothes you feel most comfortable in, which will probably be jeans. Anyone who doesn't like jeans needs counseling. ☺

There are many churches to choose from. Visit until you feel welcomed and have a sense of, "*Yes! This is it,*" felt in your heart. Here, you will be at home. You will have opportunities to learn more truths about God—and about walking with God—as you hear sermons, along with studying the Bible. This gives opportunities for loving relationships to form with other believers.

What I've come to love most is hearing the stories of what takes place in the lives of individuals once they choose to make Jesus Christ Lord of their lives. You too, can tell your story, as the Spirit prompts you, for you will indeed have a story to tell.

It is important to <u>tell others </u>of your decision to be a follower of Christ.

List the first three people you plan to tell of your decision:____

(List at least one.)

These persons may want more information, so take her or him to meet your pastor. What is also true is that you may meet with opposition. Here are two of the many verses that will help you during such times: 1 Peter 5:10, "And after you have suffered a little while, the God of all grace, who has called you to his eternal glory in Christ, will himself restore, confirm, strengthen, and establish you.

1 Peter 1:13, "Set your hope fully on the grace that will be brought to you at the revelation of Jesus Christ."

For more help, visit:

https://www.thegospelcoalition.org/article/10-ways-christians-should-respond-to-opposition/

Find Christians who can serve to "disciple you," meaning one who will meet with you when you want to talk about your "walk" with the Lord, a person who can help as you learn to give full loyalty to Jesus Christ's teachings, recorded in the first four books of the New Testament. Choose a person willing to help you learn more fully how to grow as a Christian and how to be a witness of your faith to others. If you are married to a Christian, it is best to choose someone other than your spouse to disciple you. However, you and your spouse can have great studies together, superb times of sharing about what you are learning and how you are applying these truths to your life.

I believe having faith in God and trusting that the Bible is rightfully called "God's Word" is the best help a person can get through their struggles in this life.

This work will reveal what is true. Finding truth will be a major and powerful part of your healing work. Even if you have had no former interest in reading the Bible, be assured the Biblical passages chosen for this workbook will hold power to reinforce your coming to understand yourself and your current struggles. The proof will be evident within the changes you will experience.

God Speaks!

Scriptures carry the Words of God spoken to people who committed themselves to listening. We have these, the New Testament and the Old Testament, as the truest source of what God wants to tell His people. They are ancient, hallowed books and favored above all Words that we hear personally from God. The Bible is an excellent measuring stick for determining whether or not what we believe God is speaking into our souls aligns well with the truth. When "hearing" that still voice within the soul, I ask, does this message give me peace? Do I feel loved as I hear these words? Do they uplift my soul? And, are the words in keeping with what is written in the Bible? If the answer to each of these defining questions is "yes," I trust that God has given those words to me.

It is also true that God speaks to all who will listen. The message below titled "God Speaks" is an example of listening/hearing. I write these in my journal, when received, during my prayer times throughout many years. Each time I "hear" I hold the words to a standard, asking myself, "Are these word in keeping with Biblical scriptures? Are they in keeping with the nature of God, who I have come to know through prayer and scripture reading? Do they call me to higher places in active service and behavior? And, do they bring peace?

The Bible shows readers clearly there is *"no respecter of persons"* with God. He loves each of us and will speak as we listen.[33]

In order to encourage readers to believe in the ability to hear, below is a shared entry written in my journal within a past prayer time:

"Trust Me, Beloved One. I am with you always and in all things. Watch and see how I take every step with you as you proceed. I will bring moment to moment joy to you as you sink deeper into living in 'the secret place of the Most High.'"

Abide there for the solace your soul seeks. I have much joy in store for you. Watch for it—as I have it in abundance for you. I have called you for a purpose. 'No weapon formed against you shall prosper' as you seek to let your mind be stayed in Me.'" [34]

We are meant to hear God speak to us. Doing so means we seek and enter closeness with God. Listening with intention of hearing God's direction and guidance is enhanced by having a pastor, a priest or person with credentialing as a "spiritual director" accompany you on this journey. Pastors can make referrals to certified spiritual directors. The website below, will provide names of spiritual directors in your city.

https://www.sdiworld.org/find-a-spiritual-director.

If hearing from God has already been an experience for you, feel free to write below what you believe God has spoken to you:__

---

[34] Isaiah 54:17.

My story

I have not suffered drug or alcohol addiction, but early in life, struggled with serious illnesses. I had multiple hospitalizations and came very close to death at points. Many prayed for me to get well—and still, I was sick, struggling to stay alive. I felt like a failure and thought God was disappointed in me for not measuring up to some standard I wasn't able to reach or comprehend. Here, I would like to share what brought me to Christ--and later to chaplaincy.

Once while in a Catholic hospital, when I was 18, I encountered the Sisters of the Holy Cross for the first time. Although I was not a Roman Catholic, these nuns had a profound effect on me. They came, day after day—and what power there was in their presence. They didn't talk so much, as they were good listeners. It was obvious they cared about what was happening to me.

How I was healed

Through them, *I got it.* My eyes were opened to see God differently. I came to understand that God was not like an earthly parent who could rage, be distant, authoritative—chastising in anger. Rather, I realized God is a loving, accepting, merciful Father.

In time, I understood that illnesses, losses and trauma were not a result of God being disappointed, or angry. Rather, I could finally see God as a wonderful, loving Personage who brought Jesus into the world. Given time and considerable healing around the issue of God *as Father,* I gradually developed a whole different sense of God, whom Jesus called "Father." I could see Jesus and God as having the same loving, accepting nature.

Because of this new view of God, my faith expanded. Given time, I learned that suffering truly has a "redemptive" side, although that truth did not come quickly or easily! How wonderful it is to know that God is right here with me in the midst of my struggles—pulling for me, empowering me to endure life's adversities.

I did gain my health, but only through a process that took a number of years. What that involved is covered in one of my books titled *The Chaplain is In: Journey to Health and Happiness.* There I tell more about how to let go all negatives, watch for thoughts that are not wholesome, correct beliefs that do not align with truth—and honor our emotions. For me, this is about healing my soul, as well as healing the physical tendency of my body to form blood clots which were threatening my life. In the above book I include factors explored within a new field in medical science, psychoneuroimmunology (PNI), which fully verifies how the health of the mind and emotions affect both body and soul.

One of the things I had to do was learn to forgive. This meant letting go the pain of the past. I learned that forgiving is a process. It begins with setting my will to release the person or the situation that has caused me pain. I learned to let go of it—and to give it all to God.

This took time and determination, but with persistence I gained relief from all that hurt me in the past. Forgiving those old wounds certainly affected the health of my body. Although the work was gradual, peace and joy were felt, making it like an adventure unfolding.

It was much earlier in life, however, when I encountered someone who was—and is—more important than the Roman Catholic nuns. That was Jesus. He came to my awareness at age eight, during a time when I had not heard of Him. Our family did not attend church; talk of God was not heard at home. Yet, for some reason Mom and Dad sent me to a Quaker girl's summer camp. There Jesus Christ was introduced in such a loving, caring way that my heart was deeply touched. The building where we met was called "the Tabernacle."

At the end of that first service an altar call was made. Any individuals wanting to accept Jesus into their hearts and lives were invited to go forward to kneel at the altar rail, which served to validate that decision. Love and appreciation for this Jesus came easily because of the way the speaker so aptly portrayed Him. I made my choice. Every night for the rest of the week, I walked down that "sawdust trail" to kneel at the altar. I wanted to make sure *it took*. Yet, I think those multiple trips to the altar were really about my wanting to experience more and more of that great love.

After that, outstanding changes took place in our family. My parents began attending church with my sister and me. Years later Mom and Dad became ministers at home and later traveled to expand Christ's teachings in numerous countries. Two more siblings were born, and today each one of us is doing some sort of ministry with people who are in need.

The decision I made as an eight-year-old was the most significant event of my life. God's mercy and grace have become more and more evident throughout life as I continue to place the Gospel of Jesus above all else. For sure, I have not been perfect. Yet, my goal is to stay on the path of seeking God's will over my own, day-by-day.

My life experiences, and my failures, have taught me that this is the best of all ways to live. Practices of praying, journaling and meditating on Scripture have resulted in much healing within my soul. This has reflected powerfully in my body. Majorly, I learned *life is all about how we love*! And, love is the most powerful entity in the universe!

Growth will not stop as imperfections keep coming to light. Yet, as a believer, I seek to stay in service, extending to others the kind of love I've experienced from God and from others. I live with a grateful heart, as there is no room for negativity. Every earthly experience is fodder for growth and change.

Where Does Chaplaincy Fit In? From early in life, I longed to help people who struggle with matters of the heart, as well as those who endure emotional and physical illness. Becoming a chaplain seemed the best way to do that. Yet, it was not possible to gain the credentialing needed to serve as a chaplain until my family was raised. So, during my 50's, I began Clinical Pastoral Educational (CPE), a yearlong internship in a teaching hospital. Within my training I *knew this was my call*—and that the call was clearly *worth the wait*. Chaplaincy training was followed by Board certification after which I gained a master's degree in theology.

Twenty-four years have passed, during which I have done chaplaincy in hospitals, hospice and jail settings. When Dr. Leslie Edison called a month ago saying she wanted me to counsel patients who are on Suboxone, a medication that ends cravings and withdrawal symptoms as they seek to recover from opioid addiction—I wondered if I was ready for this. The following week ministers referred two Marines for counselling. After two or three sessions, I felt confident. If my work was up to the standard these military men expected—clearly, I was ready. Onward and upward is the rule of life when we determine to be all we can be for the sake of making it a better world.

Addiction Bibliography
The Most updated helps are found online

Each site listed in the bibliography has been Accessed as recently as 5-19-2020

Many times family members or friends need a little help understanding opioid use disorder (OUD), or alcohol dependence. Watching some short Youtube videos together will provide opportunity to discuss them:

https://www.youtube.com/watch?v=SufLpGPauII

https://www.youtube.com/watch?v=TTMNXzL4O4s

See "Letters to teens" below for more good websites for family use.

*

https://www.addictioncenter.com/treatment/medications/suboxone/

This site extends information on medications prescribed most for people seeking recovery from opioid addiction. Here, Suboxone is referred to as "the preferred treatment medication for opioid addiction." Dr. Adam Bisaga, a renowned expert in opioid treatment is quoted, "When taken properly, individuals on Subonxone will have no cravings, have no withdrawal, and will feel 'normal' . . . that is why it's so effective."

*

https://www.ncbi.nlm.nih.gov/books/NBK534504/

Highly beneficial information on opioid use disorder (OUD) can be found through books published by NCBI. These are free online books presenting current information about medications that eliminate cravings and physical withdrawal symptoms for people seeking recovery from addiction. This is called medication-assisted treatment **(MAT)** and can be prescribed by health providers. The science demonstrating the effectiveness of **(MAT)** is strong.

*

https://www.nationalacademies.org/our-work/medication-assisted-treatment-for-opioid-use-disorder

An excerpt from The National Academies Sciences, Engineering, Medicine:

"The opioid crisis in the United States has come about because of excessive use of these drugs for both legal and illicit purposes and unprecedented levels of consequent opioid use disorder (OUD). More than 2 million people in the United States are estimated to have OUD, which is caused by prolonged use of prescription opioids, heroin, or other illicit opioids. OUD is a life-threatening condition associated with a 20-fold greater risk of early death due to overdose, infectious diseases, trauma, and suicide. Mortality related to OUD continues to escalate as this public health crisis gathers momentum across the country, with opioid overdoses killing more than 47,000 people in 2017 in the United States. Efforts to date have made no real headway in stemming this crisis, in large part because tools that The opioid crisis in the United States has come about because of excessive use of these drugs for both legal and illicit purposes and unprecedented levels of consequent opioid use disorder (OUD). More than 2 million people in the United States are estimated to have OUD, which is caused by prolonged use of prescription opioids, heroin, or other illicit opioids. OUD is a life-threatening condition associated with a 20-fold greater risk of early death due to overdose, infectious diseases, trauma, and suicide. Mortality related to OUD continues to escalate as this public health crisis gathers momentum across the country, with opioid overdoses killing more than 47,000 people in 2017 in the United States. Efforts to date have made no real headway in stemming this crisis, in large part because tools that already exist—like evidence-based medications—are not being deployed to maximum impact."

A free pdf of *Medications for Opioid Disorder Saves Lives* can be downloaded at **https://www.nap.edu/read/25310/chapter/1** This booklet is published by The National Academies Sciences, Engineering, Medicine.

*

https://www.youtube.com/watch?v=xdlNf_Gtq9Q

The above Youtube discusses overdose prevention for clinicians treating patients with opioids for chronic pain. It is less than five minutes long. Ideally, a patient can take an electronic tablet to his or her health provider so they can view this Youtube together. This will be educative. But also will create the best possibility of patient-centered care.

*

Opioid-bibliography-FINAL.pdf

The above site offers an extensive annotated "Opioid Bibliography." It contains 20 reference sites, each covering aspects of the current opioid crisis. Although this sophe.org site holds varied helps, the information was published in 2018 so may not contain the most up to date information. It is included, here, as an excellent source for discovering what universities, government agencies and other entities are studying addiction and, in some instances, publishing cutting edge information. Readers can use this site for seeking updates specific to individual needs and interests. For instance, if a reader is interested in alternative strategies for chronic pain care, a link is included in this Opioid Bibliography with key studies related to chronic pain treatment.

*

https://healthreach.nlm.nih.gov/document/940/Pregnancy-and-opioids-Opioid-addiction-part-10

This is a good site for identifying risks to the health of the unborn baby when a mother is on opioid drugs. It covers "birth defects, stillbirth, and premature birth, as well as withdrawal symptoms known as neonatal abstinence syndrome (NAS)."

The two SAMHSA sites below offer additional information concerning alcohol or opioid use during pregnancy:

https://store.samhsa.gov/product/Treating-Babies-Who-Were-Exposed-to-Opioids-Before-Birth/SMA18-5071FS3

https://store.samhsa.gov/product/Opioid-Use-Disorder-and-Pregnancy/SMA18-5071FS1

*

https://www.aau.edu/research-scholarship/featured-research-topics/persons-perception-risk-can-tell-us-about-their

This site extends an Association of American Universities study presented January 2020 by JAMA Psychiatry. It reveals how a person's strong tolerance to risk-taking can highly influence the potential for relapse. This website provides information about the JAMA study, but also offers a link to the study itself. The study's findings help clinicians better predict which patients are most vulnerable, but also serves to educate aspects of risk-taking for people who use opioids and want to understand the fulcrum of their triggers for using opioids.

*

https://www.mayoclinic.org/diseases-conditions/prescription-drug-abuse/in-depth/how-opioid-addiction-occurs/art-20360372

This is a site that shows how an addiction to an opioid occurs. It helps a reader understand the body's physical response to opioids. It also shows why opioids are so highly addictive. Tolerance is explained and what takes place in the body as a person feels driven to increase their doses in order to experience again feeling so exceedingly good. Here, superb information reveals why relapse often causes death.

https://www.drugabuse.gov/publications/opioid-facts-teens/letter-to-teens

"Letters to teens" covers such topics as how pain relievers, prescribed after

a sports injury can be very addictive resulting in Opioid Use Disorder (OUD)

and consequential overdoses, sometimes causing death. These additional sites are for teens that are interested in understanding OUD and want to know how best to protect their brains while growing:

https://www.youtube.com/watch?v=EpfnDijz2d8

https://www.youtube.com/watch?v=Xbk35VFpUPI

https://www.youtube.com/watch?v=YlFDDB061i8

https://www.youtube.com/watch?v=wCMkW2ji2OE

https://www.youtube.com/watch?v=IAowbBbb8YY

*

https://blog.tedmed.com/brain-in-progress-nora-volkow/

A video on which Dr. Nora Volkow, Director of the National Institute on Drug Use talks on, "Brain in Progress: Why Teens Can't Always Resist Temptation"

*

https://store.samhsa.gov/product/Opioid-Overdose-Prevention-Toolkit/SMA18-4742

This toolkit offers strategies to health care providers, communities, and local governments for developing practices and policies to help prevent opioid-related overdoses and deaths. Access reports for community members, prescribers, patients and families, and those recovering from opioid overdose may be found here: Publication ID SMA18-4742 Publication Date: June 2018

https://www.integration.samhsa.gov/integrated-care-models/toolkits
Here a wide-scope of information, including topics on "Recovering from Opioid Overdose" and "Resources for Overdose Survivors and Family Members."

*

https://newsinhealth.nih.gov/2018/10/managing-pain

The site is about managing pain while moving beyond opioids. This is very clear and helpful.

*

https://heal.nih.gov/research

NIH launched the Helping to End Addiction Long-Term (HEAL Initiative). The focus is to address the shortage of effective medications for chronic pain and other issues contributing to the opioid crisis.

This is an excellent, easy to read site on understanding how chronic pain develops. Research within this initiative extends better understanding of how acute pain becomes chronic. The above site carries current news revealing plans for making a difference in the way people suffering from OUD are treated. The Helping to End Addiction Long-term^{SM} Initiative, or NIH HEAL Initiative^{SM} is now funding hundreds of projects nationwide. "Researchers are taking a variety of approaches to tackle the opioid epidemic through "an aggressive, trans-agency effort to speed scientific solutions to stem the national opioid public health crisis. Almost every NIH Institute and Center is accelerating research to address this public health emergency from all angles."

Patient-centered care is bringing more resources for recovery and treats the whole person while suppling patients with information. This care tactic is helping people make better treatment decisions as they work with the healthcare professionals who treat them.

*

https://www.youtube.com/watch?v=X1AEvkWxbLE

Dr. Nora Volkow, director of the National Institute on Drug Use at the NIH, explains addiction as "a disease of free will." She gives an excellent explanation of the "reward circuit" that exists within drug addiction.

*

https://heal.nih.gov/research/research-to-practice/brim

In March 2020, the National Institute of Health announced granting six research awards totalling $9.4 million over three years. "These grants will study the impact of behavioural interventions for primary or secondary prevention of OUD, or as a complement to medication-assisted treatment **(MAT)**."

Behavioural interventions, such as yoga, mindfulness along with cognitive behavioural therapy are discussed at this site as ways to improve adherence to medication and improve treatment outcome, thereby reducing relapses. These behavioural interventions will no doubt make a difference for those

---

114

who are able to be consistent with them. These efforts, along with MAT, will bring better results for a lasting recovery.

A concern exists as regards many people who could benefit from these initiatives but will not receive them, due to not knowing about the availability of these behavioural interventions. This will be a great loss to the goal of ending the opioid epidemic, unless the general public along with all health providers and treatment centers are made aware of these initiatives. Without this, the success of these initiatives affecting the opioid epidemic could be greatly limited—failing to reach those needing recovery from OUD.

Currently, there is a serious lack of public awareness regarding medication-assisted treatment **(MAT)**. Medications like Suboxone or Vivitrol that control cravings and physical withdrawal symptoms need widespread publication, especially since MAT holds the greatest potential for helping people with drug dependency reach recovery.

*

https://store.samhsa.gov/product/Adult-Drug-Courts-and-Medication-Assisted-Treatment-for-Opioid-Dependence/sma14-4852

This guide includes strategies to increase the use of MAT in drug court programs.

*

https://store.samhsa.gov/product/Adult-Drug-Courts-and-Medication-Assisted-Treatment-for-Opioid-Dependence/sma14-4852

The current opioid crisis brings to the fore the great need for all treatment courts to adopt best practices related to medication-assisted treatment **(MAT)**. Updated material is needed on this matter.

*

https://www.naabt.org/documents/NAABT_Language.pdf

"Words are important. If you want to care for something, you call it a 'flower'; if you want to kill something, you call it a 'weed'." By Don Coyhis (Dedicated in loving memory of John A. Strosnider, DO.)

Stigma is a mammoth barrier to addiction treatment. The above site helps understand that terminology used to describe addiction has contributed to the stigma and offers suggestions for change.

*

Grace, Annie. *This Naked Mind: Control Alcohol, Find Freedom, Discover Happiness & Change Your Life,* (New York, Penguin Random House, 2018).

Annie does good work reviewing the truth of how for decades the alcohol industry has heavily influenced the minds of people with their ad campaigns.

Alongside that, she shows the various sources of media have present alcohol as being the elixir for well-being. Both consciously and subconsciously, many (now hooked) bought the message of alcohol being the anecdote for stress—serving up fun times by making drinkers of alcohol unique, witty, bold, courageous and sexually appealing. Who would not want all that? Grace says the ad campaigns and media's portrayal of alcohol, "promise **fulfilment**, satisfaction, and happiness." Her book clearly shows alcohol for what it is versus the hype—a highly addictive poison that does the opposite of what the alcohol industry claims. Those who use alcohol know it stultifies the brain, shuts down sensitivity along with the mental acumen needed for making adequate decisions.

Most of us have not known that alcohol impedes the immune system, renders people prone to cancer and a multitude of other diseases. Grace explains this well, while also making clear the massive societal problems that result from the use of alcohol. Grace's approach for ending alcohol addiction is ever so unique. As one reviewer, who now abstains 100%, puts it, "…as long as you pay attention, and think about what the author says, the actual change happens subconsciously." How? Because, according to this author, once the truth about alcohol is received within a person's subconscious

 mind, the mental and emotional desire for the alcohol ends. Voila! Freedom restores one's life . . . by granting freedom from the physical cravings and withdrawal symptoms and freedom from the stigma that addiction brings. Grace knows from her own experience of having been addicted to alcohol, how heavy drinking carries a super-huge price tag. The process of gaining freedom can take place in ten days after a last drink, according to Grace. If I were a drinker reading this book, I'd jump on this wagon!

My only criticism of this well-reviewed book is that medication-assisted treatment **(MAT)** is not covered well. These medications are available and can be prescribed by a medical provider. Some insurance plans cover the cost of MAT and many state programs are available for people who do not have insurance. The author also misses an opportunity to publicize the truth that these medications can end the cravings experienced while a person goes through detox on course toward recovery. Counselling helps seal the deal, actually. More could have been said by this author about the benefits of counselling. She did mention counselling, but with little emphasis.

Other books by Joy Le Page Smith

Available for purchase at Amazon.com

or from her website:

www.healing-with-Joy.com

*The Little Mountain Goat Who
Was Afraid of High Places*

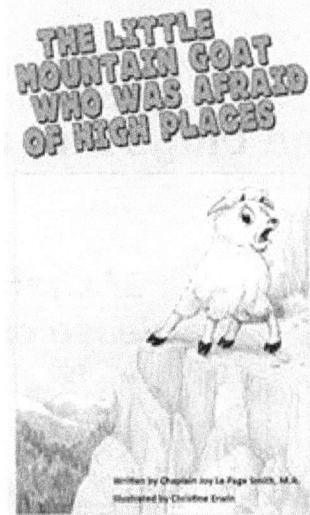

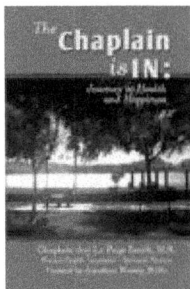

The Chaplain is In: Journey

to Health and Happiness

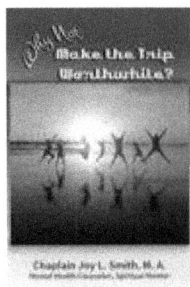

Why Not Make the Trip Worthwhile?

See additional helps at Joy Le Page Smith's website:

www.healing-with-Joy.com

***

The blogs and articles listed below are <u>free</u> to use.

If sharing from these writings below,
please credit www.healing-with-Joy.com

<u>"Quick Aids" button on website brings the following articles and prayers:</u>

Help with Granting Forgiveness

Dealing with Difficult Emotions - Finding Emotional Freedom

Tips for Teaching Children How to Identify What They Are Feeling

Are You Suffering from False Guilt

What Are You Ashamed Of?

"To Err is Human, to Forgive Divine"

Setting Boundaries within Relationships

More Help with Setting Boundaries

Inner Healing Exercise

The Best 50 Minutes of Your Life

Extra pages for notes~~

Extra pages for notes~~

www.ingramcontent.com/pod-product-compliance
Lightning Source LLC
Chambersburg PA
CBHW081418270326
41931CB00015B/3323